# Handbook of Myocardial Revascularization and Angiogenesis

# Handbook of Myocardial Revascularization and Angiogenesis

*Edited by*

**Ran Kornowski** MD
Director of Experimental Pharmacology and the Myocardial Revascularization Program
Cardiovascular Research Foundation
Washington Cardiology Center
Washington DC
USA

**Stephen E Epstein** MD
Director of Vascular Biology Research
Cardiovascular Research Foundation
USA

**Martin B Leon** MD
Chief Executive Officer and President
Cardiovascular Research Foundation
USA

MARTIN DUNITZ

© Martin Dunitz Ltd 2000

First published in the United Kingdom in 2000 by
Martin Dunitz Ltd
The Livery House
7–9 Pratt Street
London NW1 0AE

A CIP catalogue record for this book is available from the British Library

ISBN 1-85317-782-2

Distributed in the United States by:
Blackwell Science Inc.
Commerce Place, 350 Main Street
Malden MA 02148, USA
Tel: 1–800–215–1000

Distributed in Canada by:
Login Brothers Book Company
324 Salteaux Crescent
Winnipeg, Manitoba R3J 3T2
Canada
Tel: 1–204–224–4068

Distributed in Brazil by:
Ernesto Reichmann Distribuidora de Livros, Ltda
Rua Coronel Marques 335, Tatuape 03440–000
Sao Paulo,
Brazil

Composition by Wearset, Boldon, Tyne and Wear

Printed and bound in Spain by Grafos, S. A.

# CONTENTS

## II    Therapeutic myocardial angiogenesis

# Contributors

**Keith B Allen** MD
Department of Cardiothoracic Surgery
St Vincent Hospital and
The Indiana Heart Institute
Indianapolis, IN 46260
USA


**Stephen W Boyce** MD
Department of Cardiothoracic Surgery
Washington Hospital Center
110 Irving Street NW
Washington DC 20010
USA


**Didier Branellec** PhD
Rhône-Poulenc Rorer
Gencell
CRVA
13 Quai Jules Guesde
BP 14
94403 Vitry Sur Seine Cedex
France


**Daniel Burkhoff** MD PhD
Department of Medicine
Columbia University
630 W 168th Street
New York, NY 10032
USA


**Ronald G Crystal**
New York Presbyterian Hospital–Weill
    Medical College of Cornell University
525 E 68 Street
New York, NY 10021
USA


**Stephen E Epstein** MD
Cardiology Research Foundation
Washington Hospital Center
110 Irving Street NW
Washington DC 20010
USA


**Shmuel Fuchs**
Cardiology Research Foundation
Washington Hospital Center
110 Irving Street NW
Washington DC 20010
USA


**Warren S Grundfest** MD FACS
Dept of Biomedical Engineering
University of Southern California
Los Angeles, CA 90089
USA

**David R Holmes Jr** MD
Dept of Internal Medicine and
    Cardiovascular Diseases
Mayo Clinic and Foundation
200 First Street SW
Rochester, MN 55905
USA

**Dongming Hou** MD PhD
Krannert Institute of Cardiology
1111 W 10th Street
Indianapolis, IN 46202-4800
USA

**Jeffrey M Isner** MD
Tufts University School of Medicine and
St Elizabeth's Medical Center
736 Cambridge Street
Boston, MA 02135
USA

**Jim Jones** MD
Department of Medicine
Columbia University
630 W 168th Street
New York, NY 10032
USA

**Birgit Kantor** MD
Dept of Internal Medicine and
    Cardiovascular Diseases
Mayo Clinic and Foundation
200 First Street SW
Rochester, MN 55905
USA

**Ran Kornowski** MD
Cardiology Research Foundation
Washington Hospital Center
110 Irving Street NW
Washington DC 20010
USA

**Roger J Laham** MD
Harvard Medical School
Angiogenesis Research Center and
Interventional Cardiology
Beth Israel Deaconess Medical Center
Boston, MA 02215
USA

**Daisy F Lazarous** MD
The Johns Hopkins University School of
    Medicine
Division of Cardiology
The Johns Hopkins Bayview Medical
    Center
4940 Eastern Avenue
Baltimore, MD 21224
USA

**Kenneth T Lee**
New York Presbyterian Hospital–Weill
    Medical College of Cornell University
525 E68 Street
New York, NY 10021
USA

**Leonard Y Lee**
New York Presbyterian Hospital–Weill
    Medical College of Cornell University
525 E68 Street
New York, NY 10021
USA

**Martin B Leon** MD
Cardiology Research Foundation
Washington Hospital Center
110 Irving Street NW
Washington DC 20010
USA

**Douglas W Losordo** MD
Tufts University School of Medicine and
St Elizabeth's Medical Center
736 Cambridge Street
Boston, MA 02135
USA

**Edward R McCluskey** MD PhD
Genentech Inc.
1 DNA Way
South San Francisco, CA 94080-4990
USA

**Charles J McKenna** MD
Department of Internal Medicine and
    Cardiovascular Diseases
Mayo Clinic and Foundation
200 First Street SW
Rochester, MN 55905
USA

**Abder Mahfoudi** PhD
Rhône-Poulenc Rorer
Gencell
CRVA
13 Quai Jules Guesde
BP 14
94403 Vitry sur Seine Cedex
France

**Keith L March** MD PhD FACC
Krannert Institute of Cardiology
1111 W 10th Street
Indianapolis, IN 46202-4800
USA

**Stephen N Oesterle** MD
Harvard Medical School
Director, Invasive Services
Massachusetts General Hospital
55 Fruit St, Bulfinch 106
Boston, MA 02114
USA

**Thanassis Papaioannou** MSc
Laser Research and Technology
    Department
Cedars-Sinai Medical Center
Los Angeles, CA 90048
USA

**Richard Pilsudski** PhD
Rhône-Poulenc Rorer
Gencell
20 Avenue Raymond Aron
92165 Antony Cedex
France

**Todd K Rosengart** MD
New York Presbyterian Hospital–Weill
    Medical College of Cornell University
525 E 68 Street
F-2103
New York, NY 10021
USA

**Bertrand Schwartz** DVM PhD
Rhône-Poulenc Rorer
Gencell
CRVA
13 Quai Jules Guesde
BP 14
94403 Vitry sur Seine Cedex
France

**Robert S Schwartz** MD
Department of Internal Medicine and
    Cardiovascular Diseases
Mayo Clinic and Foundation
200 First Street SW
Rochester, MN 55905-0001
USA

**Carl J Shaar** PhD
Department of Cardiothoracic Surgery
St Vincent Hospital and
The Indiana Heart Institute
Indianapolis, IN 46260
USA

**Ramez E N Shehada** PhD
Dept of Biomedical Engineering
Olin Hall of Engineering, Room 500
University Park – MC 1451
University of Southern California
Los Angeles, CA 90089–1451
USA

**Michael Simons** MD
Harvard Medical School
Director, Angiogenesis Research Center
Beth Israel Deaconess Medical Center
Boston, MA 02215
USA

**Marvin J Slepian** MD
Sarver Heart Center
University of Arizona
PO Box 245037
1501 N Campbell Avenue
Tuscon, AZ 85724-5037
USA

**Fabienne Soubrier** PhD
Rhône-Poulenc Rorer
Gencell
CRVA
13 Quai Jules Guesde
BP 14
94403 Vitry sur Seine Cedex
France

**Thomas J Stegmann** MD FECTS
Department of Thoracic and
    Cardiovascular Surgery
Fulda Medical Center
Pacelliallee 4
36043 Fulda
Germany

**Gregg W Stone** MD
Cardiovascular Research Foundation
Washington Hospital Center
110 Irving Street NW
Washington DC 20010
USA

**Peter R Vale** MD
St Elizabeth's Medical Center
736 Cambridge Street
Boston, MA 02135
USA

**Robert J Whitbourn** MBBS BMedSC
University of Melbourne and
Director of Coronary Care
St Vincent's Hospital Melbourne
41 Victory Parade
Fitzroy, Vic 3065
Australia

# ACKNOWLEDGEMENTS

With projects like this, there are a great many people to whom we are indebted and whose names do not appear in the chapters: the technicians and researchers whose work in the laboratory has made possible these new technologies of direct myocardial revascularization and angiogenesis. We are grateful to the contributors for their excellent chapters and for the time they have spent ensuring that full details of the machines and genes they use are of practical use to the interventional cardiologist. Lastly, at Martin Dunitz we are indebted to our commissioning editor, Alan Burgess, for his diligence in continuing to publish interventional cardiology books and to his colleague, Clive Lawson, for guaranteeing a rapid publication schedule.

# PREFACE

Over the past 30 years, therapy for ischemic coronary artery disease has focused on conventional anti-anginal pharmacology, surgical revascularization techniques, and catheter-based angioplasty modalities. Current anti-anginal drug therapy has attempted to restore myocardial oxygen supply and demand mismatch by reducing demand side factors without importantly changing coronary blood flow or myocardial perfusion. Conversely, surgical revascularization and angioplasty are intended to improve coronary flow and myocardial perfusion in ischemic zones by restoring antegrade flow via the epicardial coronary arteries. Presently we are confronted by a growing cohort of patients who remain refactory to all standard forms of therapy with ongoing symptoms and ischemia despite best attempts to apply combinations of drugs, surgery, and angioplasty. In this setting of growing and important clinical need, the new fields of direct myocardial revascularization and angiogenesis have sprung forward and may now provide an alternative means to provide clinical benefit.

Direct myocardial revascularization is a generic term meant to embrace all forms of treatment involving intramyocardial approaches to enhance local myocardial perfusion *directly*—not via the epicardial coronary tree. Over the last 5 years, surgical and now catheter-based approaches using lasers (and other energy sources) are being studied as a new adjunctive therapy in refractory patients with ischemic coronary disease. The likely mechanism of action relates to local inflammatory changes which amplify endogenous angiogenesis to provide micro- and macrovessel formation in the form of both angiogenesis and arteriogenesis. These improved collateral pathways should change the local ischemic milieu and may be a durable treatment approach in selected patients. Since angiogenesis appears to be a fundamental mechanism associated with direct myocardial revascularization procedures, it seems natural to combine the overall field of angiogenesis therapy as part of this handbook. Angiogenesis therapy builds on the seminal observations of Folkman, proposing to deliver angiogenic cytokines to the myocardium via multiple routes, again in an effort to enhance local myocardial perfusion and achieve therapeutic benefit in hypoperfusion states.

The combined fields of direct myocardial revascularization and angiogenesis represent some of the most potentially exciting new approaches to patients with ischemic heart disease. This handbook brings together experts and pioneers in this interdisciplinary field, including molecular biologists, animal physiologists, cardiovascular surgeons, interventionalists, and others. Updated reports from preclinical animal experimental studies and both completed and ongoing clinical trials are presented to provide a comprehensive overview of rapidly changing and newly defined therapeutic treatment concepts. Clearly, if work done by these pioneering basic and clinical scientists demonstrates conclusive patient benefit by improving intramyocardial blood flow, the overall extension of these principles and therapies will apply to a vast cohort of patients with clinically important coronary artery disease.

*Martin B Leon, Stephen E Epstein and Ran Kornowski*

# I
# DIRECT MYOCARDIAL REVASCULARIZATION

# 1. CARDIOGENESIS™ SURGICAL TRANSMYOCARDIAL REVASCULARIZATION (ANGINA TREATMENTS: LASERS AND NORMAL THERAPIES IN COMPARISON: THE ATLANTIC TRIAL)

Daniel Burkhoff and Jim Jones for the ATLANTIC Investigators

## Introduction

Transmyocardial revascularization (TMR) has been proposed as a treatment option for patients who suffer from chronic angina and who are not candidates for coronary artery bypass surgery (CABG) or percutaneous transluminal coronary angioplasty (PTCA). To assess the safety and efficacy of TMR with a holmium:yttrium-aluminum-garnet (Ho:YAG) laser in patients with stable chronic medically refractory angina resulting from coronary artery disease in regions of the myocardium that are untreatable by CABG or PTCA, we undertook a prospective, multicenter, controlled randomized study, known as the ATLANTIC trial.

## The ATLANTIC trial

The ATLANTIC trial was done at 16 clinical sites in the USA. Between October, 1996, and January, 1998, 182 patients with severe medically refractory angina were prospectively randomly assigned either TMR plus continued maximal medical therapy (TMR + Meds, n = 92) or continued maximal medical therapy alone (Meds, n = 90).

The safety endpoints of the study were mortality and incidence of adverse events. The primary efficacy endpoints were angina relief and exercise tolerance. Secondary efficacy endpoints were myocardial perfusion and quality of life. Patients were assessed at 3, 6, and 12 months after treatment.

## Operative technique

Patients randomly assigned the TMR + Meds group continued to be treated with maximal medical therapy for treatment of angina and underwent the TMR procedure using the CardioSync™ TMR System (CardioGenesis Corp, Sunnyvale, CA). A limited, muscle-sparing left thoracotomy was done and transmyocardial channels were created in previously identified areas of reversible ischemia, using the Ho:YAG laser. Channels were made with a density of one channel every 1–1.5 cm². A mean of 20 ± 7.9 channels (range 9–42) was created, using an average of four bursts of laser energy to create one channel. Bleeding from most channels stopped spontaneously or with light finger pressure.

Patients randomly assigned to the Meds group continued to be treated with maximal medical therapy for treatment of angina for the duration of the study. Patients were not permitted to crossover from the Meds group to the TMR + Meds group during the 1-year participation in the study.

Echocardiography was done postoperatively to determine whether TMR treatment had any effect on global function or regional wall motion. Baseline global ejection fraction was similar in the two groups. Postoperative ejection fraction in the TMR + Meds group did not change from baseline. At 3 months, ejection fraction was also unchanged from baseline in both groups. A segmental analysis in which the heart was divided into 16 segments was also done. The postoperative evaluation identified a total of 25 segments in 81 patients, which were newly akinetic or dyskinetic. This number was similar to the results obtained at the 3-month assessment and was not significantly different from the number of new wall abnormalities detected in the Meds group at 3 months. There was no significant change in regional wall function in either group between baseline and 3 months.

## Inclusion and exclusion criteria

Patients entered into the ATLANTIC trial were representative of the general population of patients with stable, medically refractory angina who were likely to benefit from the TMR procedure. Enrollment inclusion criteria were: class III or class IV angina according to the Canadian Cardiovascular Society Angina Scale (CCSAS); maximum recommended dose of two or more antianginal medications or on the maximum tolerable antianginal medical regimen for at least 30 days; objective evidence of myocardial ischemia defined by positive dipyridamole stress test with thallium; areas of ischemic myocardium that were untreatable by CABG or PTCA; an ejection fraction of more than 30%. Exclusion criteria included unprotected left main disease of more than 70% or severe unprotected three vessel disease. A patient was judged to have unprotected left main disease or severe unprotected three vessel disease if none of the three coronary vascular territories was supplied by a patent (no lesion >50%) major vessel within the territory, or by patent previously placed coronary bypass graft inserted into a major native vessel that was also patent. Other exclusion criteria included:

hospital admission for unstable angina within the 21 days before enrolment; no angina during baseline ETT testing; chronic obstructive pulmonary disease; significant heart failure requiring diuretic dose of equivalent to more than 40 mg of Lasix daily; a history of clinically significant arrhythmias; MI within 3 months of treatment; or cardiac transplant.

# Demographics

Baseline demographic characteristics were not significantly different between the TMR + Meds group and the Meds group, except for hypertension and hyperlipidemia that were each slightly more prevalent in the Meds group. Patients in both groups had a high incidence of comorbidities and 95% had undergone at least one previous revascularization procedure. Baseline clinical status was also similar between groups.

# Results

## Mortality

There was no significant difference in mortality between the TMR + Meds and the Meds groups in the ATLANTIC trial. Fourteen patients died among the 182 randomized patients – five (5.4%) in the TMR + Meds group, and nine (10%) in the Meds group. No death was judged to have been related to the device. There was no significant difference between the survival curves for the Kaplan-Meier curves of the two groups as determined by the log-rank test.

## Serious cardiac adverse events

A total of 464 adverse events were reported in 89 TMR + Meds patients, and 274 adverse events were reported in 73 Meds patients. These events included 14 deaths and the associated antecedent events. All types of arrhythmias, the finding of left ventricular dysfunction (decrease in ejection fraction of more than 10%), myocardial infarction, and other cardiovascular events occurred with similar frequency in both groups. There was a greater incidence of serious episodes of angina resulting in a new hospital admission or prolonged hospital stay in the Meds group. Heart failure and thromboembolic disorders were reported more frequently in the TMR + Meds group. Pleural effusions, infection, cellulitis, and pneumonia occurred with a slightly increased frequency in the TMR + Meds group. Other events occurred infrequently in both groups and there was no apparent relation to the device.

# Effectiveness data

Primary evidence of the effectiveness of the TMR System was obtained by assessing angina classification (CCSAS) and exercise tolerance (ETT). Secondary effectiveness measures were myocardial perfusion (dipyridamole thallium) and quality of life (Seattle Angina Questionnaire).

## Angina class

To determine whether there was a change in the severity of angina during the study period, angina was assessed using the CCSAS at baseline and at 3, 6 and 12 months after treatment. Baseline angina class was similarly distributed between class III and class IV in both groups. For TMR + Meds patients, there was a leftward shift in the distribution of angina class, indicating a significant improvement in symptoms. This effect was present at each follow-up. For Meds patients, however, there was relatively little change in angina class distribution at any one of the follow-up points.

Although patients in the Meds group showed no significant improvement, 61% of patients in the TMR + Meds group had a two-class or greater drop in angina at 12 months. 45% of patients in the TMR + Meds group were in class I or had no angina at 12 months. TMR patients with baseline class IV angina tended to show a greater response to TMR treatment than patients with baseline class III angina: class III patients in the TMR + Meds group experienced a mean two-class drop in angina at 12 months, while class IV patients experienced a mean 2.2-class drop at 12 months.

# Exercise tolerance

To qualify for study entry, each patient had to have a minimum of two consecutive positive (limited by either symptoms or ECG criteria) exercise tolerance tests (Modified Bruce protocol) in which total exercise durations were within 15% of each other. Consecutive tests had to be done between 4 and 14 days apart, and the exercise test could not be done on the same day as the dipyridamole thallium test. Patients had to have typical angina (pain) on at least one of the two consecutive qualifying tests. Symptoms judged to be angina equivalents, such as shortness of breath and fatigue, could not substitute for pain. Patients were limited to a maximum of four ETTs in a 30-day period to meet the entry criterion.

Exercise tolerance was tested in all 182 patients at baseline. Follow-up data was available from 83 TMR + Meds patients and 78 Meds patients at 3 months, from 76 TMR + Meds patients and 76 Meds patients at 6 months, and from 74

TMR + Meds patients and 67 Meds patients at 12 months. Although patients in the Meds group had no significant improvement in exercise tolerance, exercise tolerance in the treated group improved by a significant average of 31% over baseline at 3 months, 35% over baseline at 6 months, and 34% over baseline at 12 months. The 1% change between 6 and 12 months was not statistically significant.

## Myocardial perfusion

To determine whether there was a change in myocardial perfusion during the follow-up period, dipyridimole thallium scans were performed 3, 6 and 12 months after treatment date. There were no significant differences between groups in the number of fixed defects at any of the endpoints. There was no significant difference between groups in the percentage of reversible defects as a function in change in angina class, nor was there a significant difference between groups in the change in percent reversible defects as a function of change in ETT time at month 12.

## Conclusions

Results from the ATLANTIC trial show that TMR with a Ho:YAG laser results in significant angina reduction, in significant improvement in exercise tolerance, and in acceptable frequencies of morbidity and mortality. TMR should be considered as a treatment option for patients with severe refractory angina who are ineligible for bypass or PTCA.

# 2. The Eclipse™ Ho:YAG Surgical Transmyocardial Laser Revascularization System

Keith B Allen and Carl J Shaar

## Introduction

Despite the success of current medical and surgical management of ischemic heart disease, a growing number of patients suffer from diffuse coronary artery disease (CAD) that is not amenable to coronary artery bypass grafting (CABG) or percutaneous interventions (PTCA).

Attempts at indirect myocardial revascularization, such as Beck's omentopexy (1935)[1] and Vineberg's thoracic artery implantation (1954),[2] had limited success in treating angina. In 1965, Sen proposed creation of left ventricular transmural channels for direct perfusion of ischemic myocardium with oxygenated left ventricular blood.[3] The concept of "myocardial acupuncture" was based on the reptilian heart model, and intuitive considering Wearn's 1933 description of a rich sinusoidal network present in the human heart.[4] Mirohseini and associates[5] advanced this concept by using laser rather than mechanical energy to create the channels. Subsequent clinical trials using a $CO_2$ laser showed that TMR significantly reduced angina and improved event-free survival in patients with severe angina untreatable with conventional methods.[6–9] Transmyocardial revascularization using a holmium:yttrium-aluminium-garnet (holmium) laser (Eclipse Surgical Technologies, Sunnyvale, CA) has shown similar benefits in patients with refractory class IV angina.[10–12] The clinical indications and results using a holmium laser for sole therapy in stable and unstable patients and as an adjunct to coronary artery bypass grafting (CABG) are discussed below.

## The Eclipse Holmium Laser System

The Eclipse Transmyocardial Revascularization (TMR) 2000 Holmium Laser System is a pulsed laser with a maximum energy output of 20 W (4 J/pulse). Mean clinical power output is 7 W (1.3 J/pulse) with a frequency of 5 pulses/s and a pulse width of 200 μs. The laser wavelength is in the mid-infrared (invisible) range at 2.1 μ.

Laser energy is delivered to the target tissue via a 1 mm flexible fiberoptic bundle (CrystalFlex®), allowing for both surgical and percutaneous applications. A hand piece that has an embedded CrystalFlex® fiber (SoloGrip® II) allows the surgeon to position and stabilize the laser fiber tip against the epicardial surface. Energy delivery is controlled with a foot switch and is not synchronized with the cardiac cycle; 3–8 pulses are typically required to traverse the myocardium.

## Clinical trials: TMR as sole therapy

Safety and efficacy of the Eclipse holmium laser used as sole therapy for patients with refractory angina has been assessed in two surgical trials. A prospective randomized multicenter trial compared TMR with continued medical management (MM) in stable patients with class IV Canadian Cardiovascular Society (CCS) angina not amenable to CABG or percutaneous transluminal coronary angioplasty (PTCA).[12] A parallel non-randomized multicenter trial evaluated TMR in unstable patients who were without surgical or percutaneous options and who were not able to be weaned from intravenous anti-angina medications (IVAA).[11]

### Transmyocardial revascularization versus medical management

Between March, 1996, and July, 1998, 275 patients with refractory class IV angina were prospectively randomly assigned treatment at 18 centers in the USA, and received either TMR (n = 132) or continued MM (n = 143). Enrollment inclusion criteria were: refractory class IV angina not amenable to CABG or PTCA while taking maximal medical therapy; reversible ischemia by myocardial perfusion scan within the distal two-thirds of the left ventricle; and an ejection fraction of more than 25%. Exclusion criteria included: severe chronic obstructive pulmonary disease defined as an $FEV_1$ of less than 55% of predicted value; inability to be weaned from IVAA; inability to undergo dipyridamole stress thallium scintigraphy; occurrence of a non-Q-wave or Q-wave myocardial infarction (MI) within 2 and 3 weeks, respectively; requirement for chronic anticoagulation; presence of ventricular mural thrombus; severe arrhythmias; and decompensated congestive heart failure. Baseline characteristics were similar (Table 2.1).

Study endpoints included: angina improvement defined as a reduction of two or more angina classes according to CCS definition, treatment failure defined *a priori* as death, Q-wave myocardial infarction and inability to be weaned from anti-angina medication after two attempts in a 48 h period or two or more cardiac-related readmissions to hospital; and changes in myocardial perfusion. Secondary endpoints included: frequency of cardiac-related readmission to

**Table 2.1 Baseline characteristics of participants in clinical trials using TMR as sole therapy**

| | TMR versus MM | | | Unstable patients† |
|---|---|---|---|---|
| | TMR (n = 132) | MM (n = 143) | p* | TMR |
| Age (years)‡ | 60 (10) | 60 (11) | 0.82 | 62 (10) |
| Male | 74% (98) | 76% (109) | 0.89 | 77% (114) |
| Preoperative EF (%)‡ | 47 (11) | 47 (10) | 0.88 | 48 (11) |
| Hx of CHF | 17% (22) | 26% (37) | 0.10 | 25% (37) |
| Hx of diabetes | 46% (61) | 48% (69) | 0.81 | 48% (72) |
| Hx of hypertension | 70% (92) | 71% (102) | 0.89 | 78% (116) |
| Hx of hypercholesterolemia | 79% (104) | 84% (120) | 0.42 | 78% (116) |
| Previous CABG | 86% (114) | 86% (123) | 0.92 | 82% (122) |

*The significance of differences between continuous variables and qualitative variables was determined using Student's t-test and Fisher's exact test, respectively.
†Patients with class IV angina and unable to be weaned from IVAA.
‡Mean (SD).

hospital; event-free survival (defined as freedom from death, Q-wave MI, hospital readmission for cardiac cause, or subsequent CABG or PTCA; change in cardiac medication use; exercise treadmill test (ETT) performance; and a quality of life questionnaire (Duke Activity Status Index [DASI]).

A total of 46 (32%) patients randomly assigned to MM met *a priori* defined treatment failure criteria and could not be weaned from IVAA on two attempts over 48 h. They were withdrawn from this study and rolled over (MM RO) to receive TMR under a parallel protocol for unstable patients unable to be weaned from IVAA. Thus, three patient groups were identified: those randomly assigned TMR who received TMR (n = 132), those who remained on MM throughout the study (n = 97), and MM patients (n = 46) who met treatment failure criteria and received TMR under a protocol for patients unable to be weaned from IVAA.

## Operative technique for TMR as sole therapy

Anaesthesia includes short-acting inhalation agents supplemented with low-dose narcotics and propofol. Intravenous fluids are minimized to avoid fluid overloading. External defibrillator pads are used on all patients. Patients are positioned in a 45° right lateral decubitus position and undergo a limited left anterolateral thoracotomy in the fifth intercostal space. A lower incision is always desirable since exposure of the inferior surface of the heart is difficult through a higher interspace. The pericardium is identified, and opened longitudinally and anterior to the phrenic nerve. Adhesions, when present, are divided to expose the distal two-thirds of the left ventricle. Previous bypass grafts, if still patent, are left undisturbed. Lidocaine (100 mg) and magnesium (2 g) are given before the laser portion of the case.

Laser channels are placed every cm² throughout the distal two-thirds of the left ventricle, avoiding areas that are obviously scarred. Three to five channels are placed, followed by 2–3 min of digital pressure to obtain hemostasis and allow for myocardial recovery. Epicardial ligation of a laser channel for persistent bleeding is rarely required. Intraoperative arrhythmias are unusual if channels are placed slowly and mechanical manipulation of the heart is minimized.

The laser energy, when absorbed by ventricular blood, produces an acoustic image analogous to steam that is readily visible by transesophageal echocardiography (TEE). Initially, TEE is used to confirm penetration of the laser into the left ventricle. After several procedures, tactile and auditory training enable the surgeon to confirm transmyocardial penetration without TEE. In the study described here, a mean of 30 ± 11 channels were created. Mean operative and laser times were 99 ± 13 and 25 ± 13 min, respectively.

The chest incision is closed in a routine manner. Stable patients are extubated in the operating room and transferred to the standard open-heart recovery unit. Postoperative pain management is accomplished for the first 24 h with a patient-controlled analgesia pump and ketoralac (Toradol, Roche, Nutley, NJ) and then by oral narcotics. Cardiac suppressants (β-blockers and calcium channel blockers) were avoided during the first 48 h but nitrates and angiotensin-converting enzyme inhibitors were resumed in the evening of surgery.

## Results

Perioperative mortality (in-hospital or 30-day) of TMR patients was 5% (7/132), which included one patient who died after randomization but before TMR. In the last 100 consecutive TMR cases perioperative death occurred in 2% of patients and was equivalent to the 2% (2/127) early (within 30 days of enrollment) death rate observed in MM patients who did not roll over. Patients who rolled over from the MM group, who were unstable and not able to be weaned from IVAA, had an operative mortality of 9% (4/46). Adverse events after TMR in stable patients included: ventricular fibrillation (8%), atrial arrhythmias (10%), hypotension (10%), non-Q-wave MI (5%), Q-wave MI (1%), congestive heart failure (4%), and respiratory failure (3%). Bleeding from TMR channels

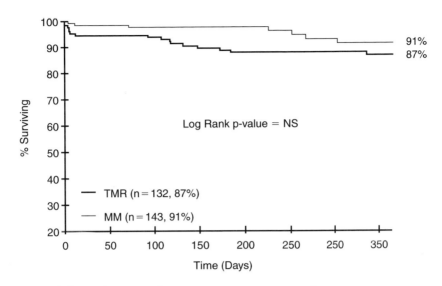

*Figure 2.1:* *Kaplan-Meier 1-year intent-to-treat survival estimates.*

requiring transfusion did not occur. At 1 year, Kaplan-Meier intent-to-treat survival estimates were not significantly different for TMR (87%) and MM (91%) patients (Figure 2.1). When MM RO patients were separated and the three treatment groups analysed, one-year Kaplan-Meier survival estimates were not significantly different among TMR (87%), MM (90%), and MM RO (91%) patients.

Significant ($p < 0.0001$) angina class improvement after TMR occurred at 3, 6, and 12 months compared with MM patients. At 12 months, 76% of TMR patients had an improvement in angina of two or more classes compared with 32% of MM patients ($p < 0.0001$). Patients who rolled over from MM and received TMR had sustained angina improvement at 12 months similar to patients observed in the TMR group (Figure 2.2). A core laboratory (Cleveland Clinic, Cleveland, OH) undertook blinded angina assessment at 12-months follow-up. A strong concordance of 80% within one angina class was observed between masked and investigator angina assessment.

Computer-quantified changes in ischemia, rest defects, and delayed defects from baseline to 12-month follow-up revealed no significant improvement of perfusion in TMR patients compared with MM patients. Since laser energy ablates myocardial tissue, there was concern that TMR might improve angina by creating zones of infarction. No differences in fixed defects were noted.

1-year Kaplan-Meier freedom from treatment failure was significantly ($p < 0.0001$) enhanced in TMR (74%) compared with MM (45%) patients (Figure 2.3). Patients randomly assigned continued MM were twice as likely to

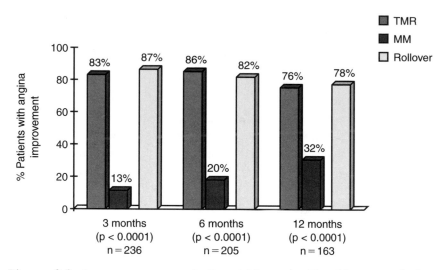

*Figure 2.2:* Angina assessment at 3, 6, and 12 months. Unstable patients had class IV angina at baseline.

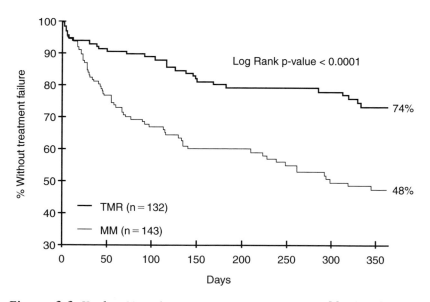

*Figure 2.3:* Kaplan-Meier 1-year intent-to-treat estimate of freedom from treatment failure.

fail therapy by 12 months compared with those who received TMR. Event-free survival (55% *vs* 31%) and freedom from cardiac-related hospital readmission (61% *vs* 33%) were significantly (p < 0.0001) enhanced in TMR versus MM patients, respectively. Using the MM RO patients as their own control, mean annualized cardiac-related hospital readmissions before TMR were 7.1 versus 0.7 after TMR (p < 0.0001).

Changes in the use of cardioactive medications (calcium channel blockers, β-blockers, and nitrates) were analysed. At 12 months' follow-up, 56% of TMR patients had decreased or discontinued calcium channel blockers compared with 24% of MM patients (p = 0.002). Likewise, β-blocker usage was decreased or discontinued in 39% of TMR patients compared with 17% of MM patients (p = 0.02). The percentage of TMR patients who decreased or discontinued nitrates was greater than that observed for MM patients, but the difference was not significant.

Improved angina and event-free survival, freedom from treatment failure, reduced cardiac-related hospital readmissions, and decreased use of cardioactive medications were reflected in better exercise tolerance (5.0 ± 0.7 *vs* 3.9 ± 0.8 METS, p = 0.05) and quality of life scores (21 ± 14 *vs* 12 ± 11, p = 0.003) in TMR patients at 12 months' follow-up.

Transmyocardial revascularization, while lacking a proven mechanism of action, offers a treatment option for patients with refractory angina who are not candidates for conventional revascularization. In this prospective, randomized, multicenter trial, stable patients with refractory class IV angina treated with TMR showed significant angina improvement, event-free survival, freedom from treatment failure, and less cardiac-related hospital readmission compared with similar patients treated with continued medical therapy.

## TMR in unstable angina

Transmyocardial revascularization in unstable patients remains controversial. March and associates[9] reported an operative mortality of 27% when treating unstable patients with a $CO_2$ laser. We hypothesized that TMR using a holmium laser in unstable patients who could not be weaned from IVAA would give significant angina relief after TMR and would have an acceptable mortality. For this study, patients were prospectively evaluated but not randomized. All patients were unstable and unable to be weaned from IVAA after at least 2 attempts in a 48 h period. Baseline characteristics are summarized in Table 2.1.

A total of 149 patients underwent laser TMR. Perioperative mortality was 11% (16/149). Significant angina improvement was observed at 3, 6, and 12 months' follow-up, with mean angina classes of 1.4 ± 1.2 (n = 125), 1.5 ± 1.3 (n = 114) and 1.6 ± 1.3 (n = 68), respectively. A limitation of this study is that all patients underwent TMR and therefore no randomized control group was used. Moreover, the natural history of these patients is not well defined, since there is no recent series of patients who had refractory unstable angina and who had medical therapy.

Transmyocardial revascularization using a holmium laser can be done with acceptable mortality in this higher-risk patient population. Improvement in angina is significant and TMR should not be denied to unstable patients who are not candidates for CABG or PTCA.

## Clinical trial: adjunctive TMR

Coronary artery bypass grafting results in incomplete revascularization due to small or diffusely diseased arteries in up to 25% of patients.[13] Incomplete revascularization adversely affects freedom from late cardiac events,[14–16] and in one series[15] was the most significant predictor of late cardiac-related deaths, angina recurrence, and myocardial infarction. In view of the success of TMR as sole therapy in patients with diffuse CAD, we hypothesized that complete revascularization by use of TMR plus CABG in patients with one or more viable target area not able to be grafted would be safe and result in a decrease in adverse cardiac events.

Between October, 1996 and October, 1997, 266 patients at 24 centers were prospectively identified whose standard of care was CABG surgery but who had one or more viable target areas not amenable to bypass grafting. Exclusion criteria included: severe chronic obstructive pulmonary disease (FEV1 < 55% of predicted value); non-Q-wave or Q-wave myocardial infarction within 2 or 3 weeks of enrollment; severe arrhythmias, and decompensated cardiac failure. Patients were randomly assigned either complete revascularization with CABG of suitable vessels and TMR to areas not amenable to grafting (n = 133), or incomplete revascularization with CABG alone (n = 133). Baseline characteristics were similar (Table 2.2).

Operative technique for CABG plus TMR included full sternotomy and CPB. The conduct of the CABG procedure and postoperative care was center-specific but not different between groups within each center. The TMR procedure was done while patients were on CPB. Operative characteristics of both groups were similar with respect to time on bypass, number and distribution of vessels bypassed, and number of endarterectomies.

Perioperative mortality (in hospital or 30 days) in CABG plus TMR patients was 1.5% (2/133) and significantly (p = 0.02) lower than the 7.5% (10/133) rate observed in CABG-only patients. Multivariable analysis of treatment group (CABG plus TMR versus CABG alone), ejection fraction, age, prior CABG, diabetes, and gender determined CABG alone as the sole predictor of operative mortality (odds ratio 5.3 [95% CI 1.1–25.7], p = 0.04). At 3 months, mortality

**Table 2.2 Baseline characeristics for TMR plus CABG versus CABG alone**

|  | TMR plus CABG (n = 133) | CABG alone (n = 133) | p* |
|---|---|---|---|
| Age (years)† | 64 (10) | 63 (10) | 0.48 |
| Male | 73% (97) | 72% (96) | 1.00 |
| Preoperative EF (%)† | 51 (13) | 50 (14) | 0.29 |
| Hx of CHF | 21% (28) | 14% (19) | 0.15 |
| Hx of diabetes | 49% (65) | 38% (51) | 0.06 |
| Hx of hypertension | 69% (92) | 79% (105) | 0.07 |
| Hx of hypercholesterolemia | 52% (69) | 64% (85) | 0.06 |
| Previous CABG | 20% (27) | 20% (27) | 1.00 |
| Predicted operative mortality‡ | 6.3% | 6.6% | 0.51 |

*The significance of differences between continuous variables and qualitative variables was determined using Student's t-test and Fisher's exact test, respectively.
†Mean (SD).
‡Parsonnet V et al. *Circulation* 1989; **79** (suppl I): 1–12.

(3% [3/117] *vs* 10% [11/115], p = 0.03) and major cardiac events (4.5% [5/111] *vs* 12.5% [15/107], p = 0.02) remained significantly lower for patients receiving complete revascularization with CABG plus TMR compared with CABG alone, with 85% follow-up. 1-year follow-up for mortality, major adverse events, angina status, and exercise tolerance is pending.

Sen[3] initially reported improved survival and decreased infarction size with mechanical TMR in an acute ischemic animal model. Mirohseini,[17] and later Horvath,[18] both using $CO_2$ lasers, observed similar results and suggested that acutely patent channels were responsible. Despite these encouraging experimental results, suggesting an acute perfusion benefit from TMR, objective evidence for acutely improved myocardial blood flow immediately after TMR remains controversial.[19,20]

This prospective, randomized, multicenter trial that compared complete revascularization with CABG plus TMR with incomplete revascularization with CABG alone shows that TMR plus CABG results in a reduction of perioperative and 3-month mortality and of major adverse cardiac events compared with

CABG alone. However, the acute benefits of TMR plus CABG in this series must be validated and long-term follow-up is still necessary.

## Conclusions

Transmyocardial revascularization by use of a holmium laser as sole therapy for stable and unstable patients with refractory angina not amenable to CABG and PTCA is safe and effective. The achievement of a more complete revascularization by use of TMR combined with CABG reduces short-term adverse cardiac events and may provide long-term clinical benefit to patients.

## References

1.  Beck CS. The development of a new blood supply to the heart by operation. *Ann Surg* 1934; **102:** 801–13.

2.  Vineberg A. Clinical and experimental studies in the treatment of coronary artery insufficiency by internal mammary artery implant. *J Int Coll Surg* 1954; **22:** 508–18.

3.  Sen PK, Udwadia TE, Kinare SG, Parulkar GB. Transmyocardial acupuncture, a new approach to myocardial revascularization. *J Cardiovasc Surg* 1965; **50:** 181–9.

4.  Wearn JT, Mettier SR, Klump TG, Zschiesche AB. The nature of the vascular communications between the coronary arteries and the chambers of the heart. *Am Heart J* 1933; **9:** 143–70.

5.  Mirohseini M, Muckerheide M, Cayton MM. Transventricular revascularization by lasers. *Lasers Surg Med* 1982; **2:** 187–98.

6.  Frazier OH, Cooley DA, Kadipasaoglu KA et al. Myocardial revascularization with laser: preliminary findings. *Circulation* 1995; (suppl II): 58–65.

7.  Horvath KA, Mannting F, Cummings N et al. Transmyocardial laser revascularization: operative technique and clinical results at two years. *J Thorac Cardiovasc Surg* 1996; **111:** 1047–53.

8.  Horvath KA, Cohn LH, Cooley DA et al. Transmyocardial laser revascularization: results of a multicenter trial with transmyocardial laser revascularization used as sole therapy for end-stage coronary artery disease. *J Thorac Cardiovasc Surg* 1997; **113:** 645–54.

9.  March RJ, Boyce S, Cooley DA et al. Improved event survival following transmyocardial laser revascularization versus medical management in patients with unreconstructed coronary artery disease. The 77th Annual Meeting of The American Association of Thoracic Surgery 1997; 94 (abstr).

10. Allen KB, Dowling RD, Heimansohn DA et al. Transmyocardial revascularization utilizing a holmium:YAG laser. *Eur J Cardiothorac Surg* 1998; (suppl 1): S100–4.

11. Dowling RD, Petracek MR, Selinger SL, Allen KB. Transmyocardial revascularization in patients with refractory, unstable angina. *Circulation* 1998; **98** (suppl II): 73–6.

12. Allen KB, Fudge T, Schoettle GP et al. Prospective randomized multi-center trial of transmyocardial revascularization versus maximal medical management in patients with refractory class IV angina: 12-month results. *Circulation* 1998; (suppl I); **98:** I-476.

13. Weintraub WS, Jones EL, Craver JM, Guyton RA. Frequency of repeat coronary bypass or coronary angioplasty after coronary artery bypass surgery using saphenous venous grafts. *Am J Cardiol* 1994; **73:** 103–12.

14. Lawrie GM, Morris GC, Silvers A et al. The influence of residual disease after coronary bypass on the 5-year survival rate of 1274 men with coronary artery disease. *Circulation* 1982; **66:** 717–23.

15. Schaff HV, Gersh BJ, Pluth JR et al. Survival and functional status after coronary artery bypass grafting: results 10 to 12 years after surgery in 500 patients. *Circulation* 1983; **68** (suppl II): II-200–4.

16. Jones EL, Craver JM, Guyton RA et al. Importance of complete revascularization in performance of the coronary bypass operation. *Am J Cardiol* 1983; **51:** 7–12.

17. Mirhoseini M, Shelgikar S, Cayton M. New concepts in revascularization of the myocardium. *Ann Thorac Surg* 1988; **45:** 415–20.

18. Horvath KA, Smith WJ, Laurence RG et al. Recovery and viability of an acute myocardial infarct after transmyocardial laser revascularization. *J Am Coll Cardiol* 1995; **25:** 258–63.

19. Landreneau R, Nawarawong W, Laughlin H et al. Direct $CO_2$ laser revascularization of the myocardium. *Lasers Surg Med* 1991; **11:** 35–42.

20. Kohmoto T, DeRosa CM, Yamamoto N et al. Evidence of vascular growth associated with laser treatment of normal canine myocardium. *Ann Thorac Surg* 1998; **65:** 1360–7.

# 3. THE HEART LASER™ $CO_2$ SURGICAL TRANSMYOCARDIAL REVASCULARIZATION SYSTEM

Steven W Boyce

## Introduction

Transmyocardial laser revascularization (TMR) is a promising new therapeutic procedure that offers relief of anginal symptoms for a growing number of patients with end-stage ischemic heart disease. There is increasing evidence for the safety and efficacy of this technique for patients who are ineligible for more traditional revascularization techniques, such as percutaneous transluminal coronary angioplasty and coronary artery bypass grafting.[1-8]

The original concept of TMR was to create transmural channels in the left ventricular free wall (LVFW) bringing oxygenated blood from within the LV cavity to the ischemic myocardium. The model for this perfusion theory is the reptilian heart with its network of sinusoids or endothelium-lined spaces in the myocardial interstitium, which serve as conduits for blood. Evolution of the TMR procedure dates back to the 1930s, when Beck performed myopexy, omentopexy, and poudrage in an attempt to promote myocardial anastomoses. Twenty years later, Vineberg experimented with implantation of the left internal mammary artery to treat coronary artery insufficiency, and in the 1960s Sen in India and Walter in Germany used needle acupuncture as the tool to apply the same principles. Use of implanted plastic tubes has also been investigated.[1,4]

These early attempts at direct perfusion had limited success since the trauma of mechanical channeling resulted in poor long-term patency of the channels. Additionally, the presence of reptilian-like sinusoids had not been documented in the human heart. These issues gave rise to the controversy that has attended heart lasers since their first use: the theory of mechanism has not been proved by histological findings, and the exact mechanism remains elusive.[5]

Due to these shortcomings, interest in direct perfusion techniques was soon eclipsed by the benefits and growing application of CABG and PTCA to bypass or widen clogged arteries. However, the increasing number of patients who are not candidates for these procedures has increased the demand for alternative treatment options.

The first use of lasers to create transmyocardial channels was by Mirhoseini and colleagues in 1981. It was thought that since laser energy vaporizes the tissue in a less traumatic way than mechanical methods, laser channels would more likely remain patent. They used a $CO_2$ laser, in combination with CABG, on an arrested heart, in that the low-powered laser was ineffective on the beating heart. The development of a higher-powered laser within the next few years, however, allowed TMR to be performed without arresting the heart, thereby obviating the necessity for cardiopulmonary bypass support and paving the way for use of the laser independent of CABG.[3]

Mirhoseini's work with animals, and then with a few selected patients, was followed in 1990 by a pilot clinical trial using the $CO_2$ laser at the San Francisco Heart Institute for 15 patients with inoperable CAD. Subsequently, a larger, non-randomized, longitudinal trial for 201 patients at eight medical centers was instituted. Other trials have since been done in the USA, Europe, and Asia. The latest outcomes are reported for 192 patients at 12 US centers, enrolled between July 1995 and September 1996, in a randomized trial comparing TMR treatment with maximal medical management.[7] All trials have noted a marked reduction in patients' anginal symptoms, an improvement in quality of life, and some increase in perfusion.

Currently, three different lasers are being used for surgical TMR: holmium:YAG, excimer, and $CO_2$. The $CO_2$ laser has been in use the longest and has the most clinical experience. To date, some 4000 patients have been treated with this type of laser, including about 2000 patients in the USA. In August 1998, the US Food and Drink Administration (FDA) approved the $CO_2$ laser for use in patients with severe stable angina untreatable by conventional techniques.

## Patients

Growing interest in TMR has corresponded with a growing population of patients for whom CABG or PTCA, the standard methods of revascularization, are not appropriate. Candidates for TMR present with severe diffuse coronary artery disease and evidence of reversible ischemia; severe angina (Canadian Cardiovascular Society class III and IV) refractory to maximal antianginal medical therapy; and coronary artery anatomy unsuitable for PTCA or CABG. Reasons for unsuitable CA anatomy include diffuse disease, inadequate distal targets, or lack of a conduit.[1,2,6]

Nearly a decade of using the $CO_2$ laser in increasingly larger trials has also helped define a subgroup of patients for whom the procedure is not recommended. As it became apparent that depressed ventricular function was the single most predictive factor of mortality and morbidity at 1 year following the procedure, a left ventricular ejection fraction of 20% or more became a criteria for laser patients in most studies. Multivariate analysis of the recently completed randomized multi-institutional trial of sole TMR treatment versus medical treatment in class III and IV anginal patients revealed that unstable angina, defined by the need for IV nitroglycerin, heparin, or both within 2 weeks of the TMR procedure, was associated with a marked increase in peri-operative mortality (27% at 1 week, 16% at 2 weeks; versus 1% thereafter).

## The procedure

A typical TMR procedure using a $CO_2$ laser takes 1 to 2 h under general anesthesia, and is done on the beating heart, without cardiopulmonary bypass support. Patients are intubated with either a single- or double-lumen endotrachial tube. A transesophageal echocardiography (TEE) probe is inserted to assess regional wall motion abnormalities and mitral valve anatomy, and to monitor myocardial function and transmural laser channel creation during the procedure. The actual laser time is approximately 20 min.[1,3,7]

With the patient in a right lateral decubitus position, a left anterolateral thoracotomy is performed between the fifth and sixth intercostal spaces. Alternatively, a thorascopic approach would use four 3 cm ports on the left side of the chest: one for the laser handpiece, one for a thorascopic monitoring system, and two for other surgical instruments. The pleural cavity is entered, the lung allowed to collapse, and any necessary pleural adhesions divided before the pericardium is opened.[3,6,7]

The pericardium is entered most commonly anterior to the phrenic nerve, and the heart is suspended in a pericardial cradle. In patients with patent disease vein grafts, care is taken to avoid manipulation which could lead to distal embolization. The ischemic myocardium, as defined by pre-operative imaging, is then exposed (Figure 3.1).[1,7]

The Heart Laser™ (PLC Systems, Inc., Milford MA) creates a TMR channel with a single $CO_2$ pulse, 30 to 50 ms in duration. It is a 1000 W instrument that delivers 800 W of power to the tissue at an energy level preselected between 10 and 40 joules. The presence of epicardial adipose tissue may require higher energy levels, as the fatty tissue tends to diffuse the laser energy. The $CO_2$ laser is aimed at the epicardium using helium-neon laser guidance, and is manipulated using a straight or 90° hand-held probe mounted on an articulated arm (Figure 3.2). The lowest energy that will create a full thickness, transmural channel, as documented by TEE, should be used to minimize postoperative diastolic dysfunction.[6,7,9] The TEE confirms transmural penetration by visualization of vapor or small bubbles, as the laser energy is absorbed by the moving blood.

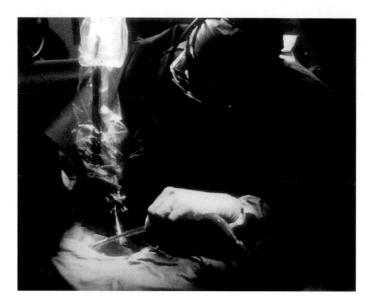

**Figure 3.1:** *A representative TMR procedure in the operating room using the Heart Laser™ CO₂ TMR system.*

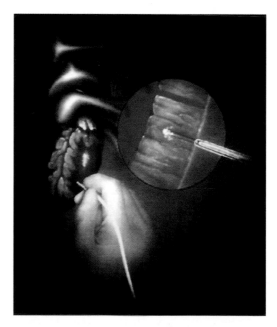

**Figure 3.2:** *A representative scheme of CO₂ channel formation using the Heart Laser™ system.*

The transmural laser channels that are created are about 1 mm in diameter and placed approximately 1 cm apart (1 per $cm^2$). In most patients, 20–30 channels are created in the LVFW. With ECG monitoring capabilities, the laser is synchronized to fire during the patient's electrocardiographic R-wave, when the left ventricle is maximally filled with blood, and the heart electrically quiescent. This timing lessens the possibility of inducing ventricular arrhythmias, and limits the risk of damage to the opposite endocardial surface or other tissues of the heart. Moving blood in the ventricle also absorbs excess laser energy.[6,7,9]

Bleeding from the laser channels is controlled by self-sealing, direct finger pressure, or, in more difficult cases, with an epicardial suture. The need for a suture is uncommon, as low as 1% in most trials. In the various studies done, patients spent about 2 days in intensive care after the procedure, and 7 to 8 days in hospital.[3,7,9]

## Outcomes

The earliest work with the $CO_2$ laser was done in patients who also underwent CABG, making it difficult to assess the independent effects of the laser procedure. In recent studies, sole therapy patients were assessed at baseline, and at 3, 6, and 12-months postoperatively for degree of angina (CCS guidelines) and quality of life. Post-TMR perfusion assessments were done with thallium or PET scanning. All trials to date have found substantial improvement in anginal symptoms and quality of life for most patients, and evidence of improved perfusion in the laser-treated areas. Specifically, in a preliminary clinical trial of 21 patients at the Texas Heart Institute, eight patients were excluded from 12-month follow-up because of death (five patients), revascularization (two), or placement of a diaphragmatic pacemaker (one). Of the remaining 13, all were free of unstable angina at 12-months' follow-up, and 11 had reduction by at least two CCS angina classifications. Mean time on the treadmill increased significantly, although there was not a significant change in mean LVEFs at rest or during stress. Mean perfusion of the treated areas increased from 45% (SD 21%) of normal at baseline to 51% (SD 23%) of normal at 12 months. Perfusion of non-laser treated areas decreased.[10]

A study of 20 patients treated from 1993 to 1995 at Brigham and Women's Hospital, Boston, USA, found all surviving patients improved from CCS class III or IV preoperatively to CCS class 0, I, or II postoperatively. There was also a significant improvement in perfusion in the laser-treated area. However, two patients died in hospital and three more after discharge.[1]

In a multi-center study at eight hospitals in the USA, 201 patients underwent TMR with the $CO_2$ laser between 1992 and 1996. Peri-operative mortality was 9% and most deaths were cardiac related. There was significant decrease in

**25**

angina class after treatment: 80% of patients dropped at least two anginal classes and 30% had no angina at all postoperatively. There was also significant decrease in perfusion defects in the treated LVFW and in hospitalizations for angina.[3,9]

In a German study, 165 patients underwent TMR between 1994 and 1997; in 20 patients, the TMR was adjunct to CABG. These latter patients were excluded from follow-up. In the sole treatment group, there was a 7.6% mortality rate. Of the survivors, 80% reported significant improvements in angina pain and lifestyle, although most thallium scans did not show significant improvement in myocardial perfusion.[4]

A randomized multi-center trial of 192 patients in the US compared TMR with continued medical management (MM). At 12-months follow-up, angina improved by at least two CCS classes in 72% of the TMR patients compared with 13% of the MM group. Quality of life improvements were also significant in the TMR group, but not the MM group. Myocardial perfusion improved by 20% in the TMR group and worsened by 27% in the MM group. Hospital admissions for unstable angina in the year after TMR were 2% for TMR patients and 69% for MM patients. Peri-operative mortality was 3% for the TMR group. That study led to US FDA approval for the Heart Laser™ in August 1998.[7]

## Mechanism

The mechanism of TMR is not completely understood, giving rise to some debate about the usefulness of the procedure despite the clear pattern of symptomatic relief reported by patients. Without histological evidence of the existence of myocardial sinusoids or of long-term patency of channels created by the laser, other hypotheses have been proposed for the mechanism of pain relief. These include: a placebo effect; a denervation effect in which the patient is unable to perceive angina secondary to nerve injury from the laser; and an angiogenic effect in which the laser causes neovascularization and thus improved perfusion and symptom relief.[2,4,11]

It is likely that several of these factors are interrelated. A placebo effect, for example, would not explain the long-term relief seen in patients 2 years or longer following TMR. On the other hand, angiogenesis would not explain the immediate relief that most patients report after TMR, although it is a logical explanation for continuing improvement in patients 3 months or longer after the procedure. Denervation may also play a role. As further experience with TMR is gained, additional insight into the exact mechanism may also be obtained.

## Current trials

The only current clinical trial with the $CO_2$ laser is the establishment of a registry for TMR patients. The registrty will monitor 600 heart laser patients (versus 'Heart Laser™'), and aims to further define the medical condition treated as well as the risk factors for peri-operative mortality and morbidity, and to evaluate the effects of operator experience on clinical results. All US medical centers with a Heart Laser™ treatment program are required to participate in the registry, which is coordinated by PLC Medical Systems, Inc.[12]

## Future directions

As the indications and applications of synergistic CABG and TMR become more fully developed and defined, the percutaneous approach is now being investigated for laser revascularization. With the catheter-based procedure, the myocardium is accessed from within the left ventricle, and the channels are created from the endocardial surface. Trials with excimer and Ho.YAG lasers are providing more information about the use of these techniques. The $CO_2$ laser, because of its wavelength, is not transmittable through fiberoptic catheters currently used, although researchers are examining ways of expanding current technology to develop such a catheter. Designs are also being developed to produce a flexible, steerable catheter able to control the 3-dimensional location of the catheter tip and the depth of ablation during TMR.[2]

Increasing knowledge of the mechanisms of TMR will lead to new and more productive uses. If laser treatment does indeed promote angiogenesis, stimulation of new blood vessel formation might be further promoted by therapy with genetic growth factors, leading to a synergistic use of the two therapies. Animal studies are currently underway to examine these possibilities.[5,13]

## Conclusion

The evidence accumulated in the past decade clearly establishes that there is a role for transmyocardial laser revascularization in the treatment of refractory ischemic heart disease. Reports by patients of angina relief and improvement of quality of life, and documentation of improved perfusion, are encouraging. As techniques are refined and further research yields more information about the exact mechanism of laser revascularization, we will better be able to apply this technology to the increasing number of patients for whom an alternative to traditional procedures is needed.

# References

1.  Horvath KA, Manning F, Cummings N et al. Transmyocardial laser revascularisation: operative techniques and clinical results at two years. *Thorac Cardiovasc Surg* 1996; **111:** 1047–53.

2.  Frazier OH, Kadipasaoglu KA, Cooley DA. Transmyocardial laser revascularization, does it have a role in the treatment of ischemic heart disease? *Tex Heart Inst J* 1998; **25:** 24–9.

3.  Horvath KA. Transmyocardial laser revascularization. In: *Advances in Cardiac Surgery*, vol. 10. St Louis; Mosby, 1988: 141–55.

4.  Krabatsch T, Tambeur L, Lieback E et al. Transmyocardial laser revascularisation in the treatment of severe diffuse coronary artery disease. In: *Transmyocardial Laser Revascularisation*. Klein M, Schulte HD, Gams E (eds). Berlin; Springer, 1998; 177–86.

5.  Narins CR, Topol EJ. Angiogenesis and transmyocardial revascularizaton. In: *Textbook of Cardiovascular Medicine Updates*. Cedar Knolls NJ; Lippincott Williams & Wilkins Healthcare, 1998; **1:**3.

6.  Smith JA, Dunning JJ, Pary AJ et al. Transmyocardial laser revascularization. *J Card Surg* 1995; **10:** 569–72.

7.  Frazier OH, Horvath KA, March RJ et al. Angina relief and perfusion improvement in patients with end-stage coronary artery disease treated by transmyocardial CO$_2$ laser revascularization: results of a prospective, randomized, controlled trial. 1999, in press.

8.  Stubbe H-M. Transmyocardial laser revascularisation with the CO$_2$ laser. In: *Transmyocardial Laser Revascularisation*. Klein M, Schulte HD, Gams E (eds). Berlin; Springer, 1998: 167–76.

9.  Horvath KA, Cohn LH, Cooley DA et al. Transmyocardial laser revascularization: results of a multicenter trial with transmyocardial laser revascularization used as sole therapy for end-stage coronary artery disease. *J Thorac Cardiovasc Surg* 1997; **113:** 645–54.

10. Cooley DA, Frazier OH, Kadipasaoglu KA et al. Transmyocardial laser revascularization: clinical experience with twelve-month follow-up. *J Thorac Cardiovasc Surg* 1996; **111:** 791–9.

11. Hughes GC, Lowe JE, Kypson AP et al. Neovascularization after transmyocardial laser revascularization in a model of chronic ischemia. *Ann Thorac Surg* 1998; **66:** 2029–36.

12. PLC Medical Systems, Inc. Post-market registry protocol summary. 1998.

13. Sayeed-Shah U, Mann MJ, Martin J et al. Complete reversal of ischemic wall motion abnormalities by combined use of gene therapy with transmyocardial laser revascularization. *J Thorac Cardiovasc Surg* 1998; **116:** 763–9.

# 4. PERCUTANEOUS MYOCARDIAL REVASCULARIZATION USING RADIOFREQUENCY ENERGY

Birgit Kantor, Charles J McKenna, David R Holmes Jr and Robert S Schwartz

## Introduction and background

Current therapy for myocardial ischemia relies on invasive revascularization procedures of the epicardial coronary arteries, or on drugs to reduce myocardial oxygen demand. There is a demand for alternative anti-anginal therapies for an increasing number of patients with advanced coronary artery disease, whose symptoms remain despite maximal treatment. Surgical transmyocardial laser revascularization (TMR) appears to be effective in treating angina.[1–5] More recently, the procedure has been done in the cardiac catheterization laboratory from the endocardial surface (percutaneous myocardial revascularization [PMR], direct myocardial laser revascularization [DMR]).[6,7] The exact mechanisms underlying the clinical success of the procedure are still unclear.[8–13]. Direct perfusion of laser channels from the left ventricle and myocardial neovascularization are the most frequently proposed hypotheses.[8,11,14,15] Other suggested explanations for the clinical benefit include an analgesic effect by denervation, a placebo effect, or a combination of these mechanisms.

It is questionable whether tissue changes after DMR and the clinical success of the procedure are specific for the laser. There is increasing evidence that energy sources other than the laser result in comparable acute and chronic pathology.[16–19] In the era of cost containment it seems desirable to have access to a safe yet more cost-efficient DMR system. We have therefore developed a new catheter-based technique to create channels from the left ventricular cavity into the endocardial surface using radiofrequency (RF) energy.[16,20–23] In this chapter, we will discuss this new DMR system and the first preclinical results.

## Is RF-PMR similar to laser TMR?

It is important to reduce the primary and secondary costs of the procedure itself, and the complications of surgery and anesthesia. In collaboration with Boston

Scientific/SciMED Inc., we have developed a safe and cost-efficient DMR approach using catheter-based radiofrequency energy, which results in very similar histological findings as laser TMR.[16,21,22]

Several investigators have suggested that acute channel morphology is key to the clinical benefit of the procedure, assuming that channels remain patent to conduct arterial blood into ischemic myocardium. Some researchers emphasized differences in acute tissue responses associated with the use of different laser systems. Investigators thought that these translate into significant differences in clinical outcome of the procedure.[24–27]

However, with increased recognition that channels do not conduct blood,[10,15] it is questionable whether the anti-anginal effect of TMR is confined to a specific energy type. Although there are differences in the immediate tissue responses associated with the various DMR approaches, it is unlikely that they translate into significant differences in long-term clinical outcome.

Typical histological findings immediately after laser DMR include intramyocardial haemorrhage and an inflammatory cell response around a thrombosed channel[28] (Figure 4.1). The blood clot that fills the wound initially serves as a provisional stroma into which inflammatory cells migrate. Blood components and inflammatory products are major sources of angiogenic growth factors. Chronically, a highly vascular scar replaces the original treatment site (Figure 4.2). The granulation tissue forming late after DMR is hypoxic, which triggers neovascularization, especially in the border zone between treated and untreated myocardium.

We have found identical histological features after radiofrequency PMR in pigs[16,22] (Figures 4.3 and 4.4). Within hours of the procedure, RF-PMR channels fill with platelets, leukocytes, and erythrocytes trapped in a fibrinous network. Chronically, a fibrous scar with a dense, blood-filled capillary network replaces the original channel site. High macrophage activity is also evident in the granular tissue up to 2 weeks after the procedure. Chronically, all channels are occluded, and both injury methods show distinct signs of angiogenesis at the previous sites of channel creation.

All DMR methods available to date cause chronic neovascularization.[28,29] As early as 1969, Hershey and White reported capillary proliferation 3 months after mechanical myocardial revascularization done with acupuncture needles. The histological appearance was similar to chronic findings after modern laser TMR and RF-PMR.[19] Recently, Malekan and colleagues[29] compared laser TMR with mechanical TMR using a power drill – the degree of neovascularization was independent of the injury method used.

However, several other studies show that heat is a crucial factor that may further enhance the angiogenesis compared with the response after mechanical channel creation.[25] Mack and colleagues compared channels created by the excimer laser with mechanically induced channels in normal sheep hearts. At 30 days,

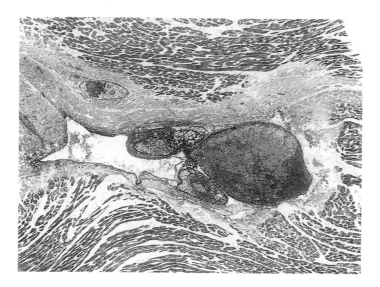

**Figure 4.1:** *Acute effects of transmyocardial laser revascularization in a patient who died 1 day after laser TMR. There are extensive blood filled spaces in the neighborhood of thrombosed TMR channels. HE, magnification × 55.*

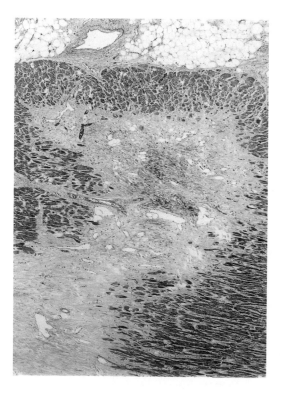

**Figure 4.2:** *Chronic findings after laser TMR in a patient who died 1 year after the procedure. The original treatment site is healed as highly vascular scar. HE, magnification × 40.*

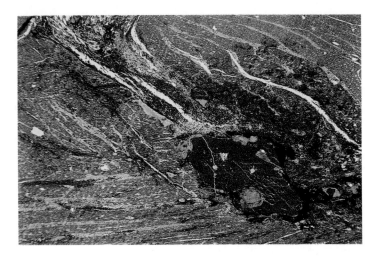

**Figure 4.3:** *Immediately after RF-PMR channels are occluded by thrombus in porcine myocardium. There is extensive intramyocardial hemorrhage around the channel site. Same myocardial appearance 1 h after RF-PMR as immediately after laser TMR as shown in Figure 5.1. HE, magnification × 48.*

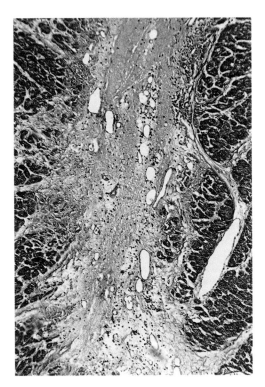

**Figure 4.4:** *Chronic findings 28 days after RF-PMR in normal porcine myocardium. The channels are healed as highly vascular scar. There is an increase of capillary density in the treated areas representing angiogenesis. Identical chronic findings after RF-PMT and laser TMR. HE, magnification × 48.*

laser treated myocardium caused a significantly higher angiogenic response than mechanical channels (2.5 ± 0.1 *vs* 1.0 ± 0.1; p < 0.5 graded on a 0 to 3 scale) suggesting that heat ablation may be an additional stimulus of angiogenesis.

Yamamoto and colleagues compared the normal angiogenic response to ischemia with the degree of neovascularization after laser TMR in a canine model.[15] Vascular proliferation assessed by bromodeoxyuridine incorporation and proliferating cell nuclear antigen was four times greater in the TMR group than the control group (p < 0.001), indicating that laser TMR was a stronger stimulus for angiogenesis than ischemia., In the next few years, data from several randomized trials will become available to give a better assessment of the efficacy and durability of the clinical benefit of DMR systems using different energies.

# Procedure and device description

Radiofrequency-PMR is done in the catheterization laboratory via a standard femoral artery access without general anaesthesia. A left ventriculogram and coronary angiogram at the beginning of the procedure show the left ventricular anatomy relevant for safe treatment.

The RF-PMR system (Boston Scientific/SciMED) consists of a radiofrequency energy generator (ArthroCare, Sunnyvale, CA), a steerable delivery catheter, and an electrode catheter. The instrumentation is easy to handle and considerably less bulky than typical laser catheters. The 9F steerable catheter and the 4.5F electrode are delivered retrograde across the aortic valve over a standard 0.035" J wire and placed in the left ventricular cavity. Radio-opaque marker bands at the distal tip of the catheters ensure fluoroscopic visibility of the catheter system.

The steerable catheter system is based on the Polaris™ (P920047/S008) family of steerable electrophysiology catheters produced by EP Technologies Inc. A stainless-steel pull wire runs the length of the catheter from the handle tip. Manipulation of the handle changes the tension on the pull wire, which deflects the distal catheter tip from 0° to 180°. The steerable system allows access to the endocardial surface of the entire left ventricle including the septum, which cannot be treated during the surgical TMR approach (Figure 4.5). When the electrode touches the endocardium, the operator activates a foot switch for the RF generator, which energizes the Nitinol electrode and support wire that serve as the electrical conduction path for the RF energy. The RF generator console operates on standard 110/220 V alternating current. It generates and controls the RF energy and the event duration. Each depression of the foot pedal results in a 0.6 s pulse of pure sine-wave energy to the electrode (465 kHz, 35 W). A ground pad, attached to the patient and connected to the generator, completes the electrical circuit and allows safe and precise energy delivery to the treatment

**33**

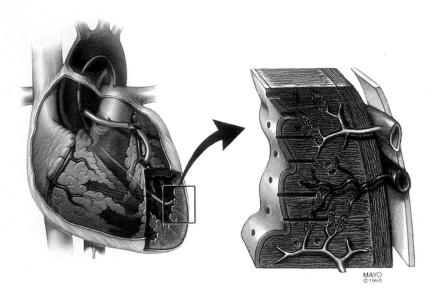

**Figure 4.5:** *Percutaneous RF-PMR can be done in the catheterization laboratory via standard femoral artery access without general anesthesia. A steerable catheter and energy delivery catheter are delivered retrogradely across the aortic valve. The steerable catheter allows access to the entire endocardial surface of the left ventricle. When the energy delivery catheter is in contact with the endocardium, channels are created by RF-ablation. The channels cause intramyocardial hemorrhage by transsecting the microvasculature (Reproduced with permission from Kantor et al. Mayo Clin Proc 1999; **74**: 585–92).*

site. A ceramic hood at the distal tip of the electrode controls lesion depth and prevents transmural myocardial penetration.

The electrode catheter has two inner lumens with ports at its tip, allowing fluid injections into the channel during the procedure. After each ablation, contrast agent is applied into the channel to mark treated sites. The contrast infiltrates the tissue and a radio-opaque blush appears on the monitor marking the channel. This provides a map of treatment sites as the procedure progresses, thereby minimizing the risk of ventricular perforation by the ablation of the same myocardial area twice. The injection port of the RF-PMR catheter can also be used for additional drug delivery of growth factors or gene therapy expressing pharmacologically active proteins to enhance the desired clinical effect of the procedure.

# Safety, morbidity, mortality

After publication of the first TMR trials it is increasingly clear that surgical TMR carries a perioperative risk of about 6–10%.[30,31] To avoid the morbidity and mortality associated with open chest surgery and general anaesthesia in the high-risk patients currently enrolled in clinical DMR trials, the RF-PMR system is only available as an interventional device for use in the cardiac catheterization laboratory. PMR has the same relatively low risk as standard procedures in the catheterization laboratory, including adverse reactions to contrast agents, stroke, and local vascular complications. Preliminary clinical studies using a similar approach in combination with laser energy show zero mortality and a very low morbidity rate.[6]

There is a 1% risk of myocardial perforation and subsequent cardiac tamponade during the percutaneous approach, since the pericardium remains intact.[22,32] This risk can be eliminated by creating shallow injuries (craters) instead of deep channels. Both approaches result in identical acute tissue responses and similar neovascularization. Ablating only the endocardial surface also minimized the relatively low risk of arrhythmia including ventricular fibrillation.[22] Thus, it is unnecessary to synchronize energy delivery to the QRS complex.

In general, these approaches are sufficient to ensure a safe procedure. Another way to reduce the risk of myocardial perforation is in-vivo tissue characterization by real-time echocardiographic imaging during the intervention. We have recently used a new high-resolution intracardiac echocardiographic catheter to improve guidance of the electrode during the procedure.[33] Imaging of the entire contracting ventricle during PMR helps to avoid the valve including leaflets, the papillary muscle, and thinned infarcted zones. The echo catheter also verifies successful radiofrequency ablation, detectable by immediate echobrightening of the treatment zone. Verifying successful channel creation in desired myocardial areas increases the success rate of the procedure.

The RF-PMR system will enter phase I clinical trial by July 1999. Early data on safety and feasibility of the procedure in patients will be available by the end of 1999.

# Physiological aspects – effect on myocardial perfusion

Radiofrequency catheter ablation has been successfully used to treat patients with cardiac tachyarrhythmias. Tissue reactions after myocardial RF ablation have been shown.[34,35] In the acute lesion, which is considerably larger than the RF channel, myocardial blood flow is diminished, as shown by contrast echocardiography.[34]

**35**

Similarly, most investigators report no improved perfusion immediately after direct laser revascularization.[10,36,37] Chronically, however, perfusion studies frequently show enhanced blood flow in treated areas.[8,15,38]

After electrophysiological RF ablation of arrhythmogenic foci, conduction occasionally recovers weeks after an initially successful ablation. The underlying mechanism for this delayed effect is not fully understood. The initial injury appears transient, leading to restoration of regional perfusion function.[34] Pathology late after RF energy application to the myocardium such as RF-PMR shows significant neovascularization, which may cause the gradual recovery of conduction and function, indicating that the newly formed blood vessels are functionally meaningful.

The limited spatial resolution of two-dimensional imaging makes it difficult to analyze the complex three-dimensional architecture and the collateralizing connections of the newly formed vascular networks. In addition, attempts to show increased perfusion late after DMR have shown conflicting results.

We use a new microscopic imaging technique (Micro-CT) to quantify and visualize complex microvascular structures. This technique enables the course of arterial blood supply from the epicardial arteries to the area of angiogenesis to be followed. After RF-PMR, three-dimensional microscopic imaging showed direct connections between epicardial coronary arteries, intramyocardial vessels, and the newly developed anastomosing capillary network in the RF-PMR treated regions.[20–22] These data show that the angiogenic region after RF-PMR connects to the surrounding myocardial vasculature, thus potentially enhancing local perfusion.

Phase I and II clinical trial, using the RF-PMR system will assess myocardial perfusion after RF-PMR in patients.

## Conclusion

Direct myocardial revascularization appears to be successful in treating angina. During the past few years, laser DMR has emerged as a therapeutic option for a growing number of patients with symptoms with end-stage coronary artery disease. Although the mechanisms behind the success of this new therapy are not fully elucidated, it may be worthwhile weighing the costs of the procedure against the costs saved by improved anginal and clinical status leading to less hospital admissions. For the high-risk group of DMR patients, the safest and most cost-effective approach should be chosen.

Using radiofrequency energy in a catheter-based technique for channel creation is a new DMR method that fulfills these criteria. Acute and chronic tissue responses after RF-PMR are identical to histological findings early and late after laser TMR, suggesting similar efficacy in patients.

Future applications for the Aries™ Radiofrequency system include RF-PMR for patients with symptoms of diffuse coronary artery disease, and RF-PMR as an adjunct to percutaneous intracoronary revascularization or incomplete coronary-artery-bypass-grafting. Since there is increasing evidence that chronic angiogenesis is a key factor in the clinical success late after the procedure, RF-PMR in combination with angiogenic factors will be investigated to further enhance perfusion.

In the next 2 years, data from the first clinical trials will be available to provide an assessment of the efficacy and durability of the clinical benefit of the new Aries™ Radiofrequency PMR system.

## *References*

1.   Cooley DA, Frazier OH, Kadipasaoglu KA et al. Transmyocardial laser revascularization: clinical experience with twelve-months follow-up. *J Thorac Cardiovasc Surg* 1996; **111:** 791–9.

2.   Horvath KA, Cohn LH, Cooley DA et al. Transmyocardial laser revascularization: results of a multicenter trial with transmyocardial laser revascularization used as sole therapy for end-stage coronary artery disease. *J Thorac Cardiovasc Surg* 1997; **113:** 645–54.

3.   Malik FS, Mehra MR, Venturo HO et al. Transmyocardial laser revascularization provides a unique and effective intervention for symptomatic relief and improvement of myocardial perfusion in diffuse cardiac allograft vasculopathy. *Am J Cardiol* 1997; **80:** 224–5.

4.   Milano A, Pratali S, Tartarini G et al. Early results of transmyocardial revascularization with a holmium laser. *Ann Thorac Surg* 1998; **65:** 700–4.

5.   Vincent JG, Bardos P, Kruse J, Maass D. End stage coronary disease treated with the transmyocardial $CO_2$ laser revascularization: a chance for the "inoperable" patient. *Eur J Cardiothorac Surg* 1997; **11:** 888–94.

6.   Oesterle SN, Reifart NJ, Meier B et al. Initial results of laser-based percutaneous myocardial revascularization for angina pectoris. *Am J Cardiol* 1998; **82:** 659–62.

7.   Yano OJ, Bielefeld MR, Jeevanandam V et al. Prevention of acute regional ischemia with endocardial laser channels. *Ann Thorac Surg* 1993; **56:** 46–53.

8.   Donovan CL, Landolfo KP, Lowe JE et al. Improvement in inducible ischemia during dobutamine stress echocardiography after transmyocardial laser revascularization in patients with refractory angina pectoris. *J Am Coll Cardiol* 1997; **30:** 607–12.

9.   Hardy RI, James FW, Millard RW, Kaplan S. Regional myocardial blood flow and cardiac mechanics in dog hearts with $CO_2$ laser-induced intramyocardial revascularization. *Basic Research Cardiol* 1990; **85:** 179–97.

10. Kohmoto T, Fisher PE, Gu A et al. Does blood flow through holmium:YAG transmyocardial laser channels? *Ann Thorac Surg* 1996; **61:** 861–8.

11. Kohmoto T, Fisher PE, Gu A et al. Physiology, histology, and 2-week morphology of acute transmyocardial channels made with a $CO_2$ laser. *Ann Thorac Surg* 1997; **63:** 1275–83.

12. Kornowski R, Hong MK, Leon MB. Current perspective on direct myocardial revascularization. *Am J Cardiol* 1998; **81:** 44E–48E.

13. Kwong KF, Kanellopoulos GK, Nickols JC et al. Transmyocardial laser treatment denervates canine myocardium. *J Thorac Cardiovasc Surg* 1997; **114:** 883–90.

14. Horvath KA, Smith WJ, Laurence RG et al. Recovery and viability of an acute myocardial infarct after transmyocardial laser revascularization. *J Am Coll Cardiol* 1995; **25:** 258–63.

15. Yamamoto N, Kohomoto T, Gu A et al. Angiogenesis is enhanced in ischemic canine myocardium by transmyocardial laser revascularization. *J Am Coll Cardiol* 1998; **31:** 1426–33.

16. McKenna CJ, Ellis L, Kwon HM et al. Identical histologic results of transmyocardial revascularization by epicardial $CO_2$ laser and endocardial radiofrequency energy: a comparison of angiogenesis in patients with a porcine model. *Circulation* 1997; **96:** I-127.

17. Malekan R, Reynolds CA, Kelley ST et al. Angiogenesis in transmyocardial laser revascularization: a nonspecific response to injury. *Circulation* 1997; **96:** I-564.

18. Whittaker P, Rakusan K, Kloner RA. Transmural channels can protect ischemic tissue: assessment of long-term myocardial response to laser- and needle-made channels. *Circulation* 1997; **93:** 143–52.

19. Hershey JE, White M. Transmyocardial puncture revascularization. *Geriatrics* 1969; **12:** 101–8.

20. McKenna CJ, Kwon HM, Ellis L et al. Microscopic 3D-CT imaging after catheter-based channel creation in normal porcine myocardium and histologic comparison with ischemic human myocardium previously treated with surgical transmyocardial revascularization. *J Am Coll Cardiol* 1998; **31:** 164-A.

21. Kantor B, Kwon H, McKenna C et al. 3-D Micro-CT: a new method for 3-dimensional rendering of myocardial channels and the microcirculation after percutaneous radiofrequency myocardial revascularization. *Zeitschrift für Kardiologie* 1998; **87** (suppl 2): 79.

22. Kantor B, McKenna C, Ritman E et al. Does channel depth affect chronic outcome after catheter-based myocardial revascularization? A histologic and 3D-microcomputed tomography study. *J Am Coll Cardiol* 1999; **33** (suppl 2A): 333A.

23. Kantor B, McKenna C, Caccitolo J et al. Transmyocardial revascularization: current and future role in the treatment of coronary artery disease. *Mayo Clinic Proc* 1999; **74:** 585–92.

24. Frazier OH, Cooley DA, Kamuran AK et al. Myocardial revascularization with laser: preliminary findings. *Circulation* 1995; **92** (suppl II): II-58–65.

25. Mack CA, Magovern CJ, Hahn RT et al. Channel patency and neovascularization after transmyocardial revascularization using an excimer laser: results and comparisons to nonlased channels. *Circulation* 1997; **96** (suppl II): II-65–9.

26. Mirhoseini M, Shelgikar S, Cayton MM. Clinical and histological evaluation of laser myocardial revascularization. *J Clin Laser Med Surg* 1990; **9:** 73–8.

27. Fisher PE, Kohmoto T, DeRosa CM et al. Histologic analysis of transmyocardial channels: comparison of $CO_2$ and holmium:YAG lasers. *Ann Thorac Surg* 1997; **64:** 466–72.

28. Gassler N, Wintzer HO, Stubbe HM et al. Transmyocardial laser revascularization: histological features in human nonresponder myocardium. *Circulation* 1997; **95:** 371–5.

29. Malekan R, Narula N, Kelley ST et al. Transmyocardial laser revascularization provides a unique and effective intervention for symptomatic relief and improvement of myocardial perfusion in diffuse cardiac allograft vasculopathy. *Circulation* 1998; **98:** II-62–9.

30. Burns S, Sharples L, Tait S et al. The transmyocardial laser revascularization international registry report. *Eur Heart J* 1999; **20:** 31–7.

31. Hughes G, Landolfo K, Lowe J et al. Perioperative morbidity and mortality after transmyocardial laser revascularization: incidence and risk factors for adverse events. *J Am Coll Cardiol* 1999; **33:** 1021–6.

32. Oesterle SN, Schuler G, Lauer B, Reifart N. Percutaneous myocardial laser revascularization: initial human experience. *Circulation* 1997; **96:** I-218.

33. Kantor B, Bruce C, Miyauchi K et al. A novel high-resolution intracardiac echocardiographic catheter improves guidance of percutaneous myocardial revascularization. *Am J Cardiol* 1998; **82** (suppl 7:A): 17 S.

34. Nath S, Whayne J, Kaul S et al. Effects of radiofrequency catheter ablation on regional myocardial blood flow. *Circulation* 1994; **89:** 2667–72.

35. Nath S, Haines DE. Biophysics and pathology of catheter energy delivery systems. *Prog Cardiovasc Dis* 1995; **37:** 185–204.

36. Kohmoto T, Uzun G, Gu A et al. Blood flow capacity via direct acute myocardial revascularization. *Basic Res Cardiol* 1997; **92:** 45–51.

37. Whittaker P, Kloner RA, Przyklenk K. Laser-mediated transmural myocardial channels do not salvage acutely ischemic myocardium. *J Am Coll Cardiol* 1993; **22:** 302–9.

38. Horvath K, Cohn L, Cooley D et al. Functional improvement, long term survival and angina relief after transmyocardial revascularization with a $CO_2$ laser. *Circulation* **98** (suppl): I-127 (abstr).

# 5. MECHANICAL MYOCARDIAL CHANNELING: A MECHANICAL ALTERNATIVE TO LASER TMR

Marvin J Slepian

## Introduction

Therapeutic management of the patient with advanced coronary artery disease (CAD) is a major challenge for the cardiologist and cardiac surgeon. Advanced CAD patients typically are symptom-limited with frequent recurrent angina, angina at low work thresholds, breathlessness, and other debilitating symptoms. For many of these patients, surgical and interventional options have either been exhausted or will result in only partial revascularization. Therapy for these patients therefore remains limited to use of multiple antianginal medications, reduction in activity, exertion, and stress levels, and significant alteration and limitation of lifestyle. Recently, significant development has been made in alternative revascularization therapies, in an attempt to provide practical stand-alone or adjunctive therapies to aid these patients. At the centre of this development is the technique of transmyocardial revascularization (TMR).

Transmyocardial revascularization, or the therapeutic revascularization of the myocardium through the creation of multiple transmyocardial physical channels, is a technique that has emerged from multiple early attempts at developing means of direct myocardial revascularization. In 1968, Sen[1] described creation of multiple mechanical punctures of the myocardial wall in a technique referred to as "myocardial acupuncture". Other investigators, including Goldman,[2] Kahzei,[3] and White,[4] also described direct myocardial needle puncturing with the vision of direct ventricular-myocardial blood communication. The goal of these efforts was to "dedifferentiate" the myocardium mechanically, creating a more reptilian substrate that uses sinusoidal blood exposure for myocardial perfusion. In 1981, Mirhoseini[5] pioneered the successful creation of substantive transmyocardial channels with the use of a laser. These and other early studies were major advances in that they provided the seminal vision and demonstration of proof of principle that clinical direct myocardial revascularization was feasible as an alternative and perhaps as an adjunctive therapy for advanced CAD. Subsequent technological improvements have allowed these early efforts to be translated into actual clinical therapy. Currently, there are three forms of laser energy TMR systems in experimental or clinical use. Recent clinical trials have shown the therapeutic efficacy of TMR, which successfully reduces clinical angina score, the number of hospital admissions for angina, and the use of antianginal medication, and augments regional perfusion and improves the quality of life for advanced CAD patients.[6–9]

Despite the promise and early clinical success of laser TMR, to date several major challenges remain. Creation of channels via laser energy carries a significant pathobiological burden. Laser channel formation may significantly damage the myocardium at the site of energy application and at distant regions.[10] Absorption of laser energy by the myocardium results in local heating and thermal damage.[10–12] Laser-mediated ablation results in severe cavitation, with generation of microbubbles and embolic debris that may have systemic embolic consequences, including stroke.[10,13] From the perspective of health-care cost, laser TMR is an expensive procedure with significant capital costs.[14,15] Laser devices are also cumbersome and require substantial maintenance and upkeep.

To address many of these limitations, an alternative means of direct myocardial revascularization has been developed, known as mechanical myocardial channeling (MMC).[16,17] MMC creates channels, either transmural or partial thickness, in the myocardium, by use of mechanical rather than laser energy. MMC combines rotary coring with vacuum tissue extraction to create clean, discrete channels with controlled degrees of myocardial injury. The rationale behind this approach was threefold: to overcome experimental and clinically demonstrated limitations of laser TMR; to develop a therapeutic approach that would allow for independent manipulation of therapeutic variables and mechanisms that contribute to the chronic improvement observed after direct revascularization; and to develop a platform technology to allow for pharmacological, cellular, and genetic therapies to be integrated for therapeutic synergy.

This chapter describes and discusses the method and devices of myocardial channeling, and recently completed experimental studies are reviewed. Eight questions are addressed: 1. What are the limitations of laser TMR? 2. What is mechanical myocardial channeling? 3. What devices may be used for MMC? 4. How does MMC simplify direct revascularization and overcome the limitations of laser TMR? 5. What are the acute whole animal and myocardial responses to transmyocardial mechanical channeling (TMC)? 6. What are the chronic myocardial healing responses to TMC? 7. Does the strategy of "TMC + healing" limit ischemic consequences of acute coronary occlusion? 8. How might MMC be combined with pharmacological and biological therapies for enhanced angiogenesis and vasculogenesis?

# What are the limitations of laser TMR?

Although direct myocardial revascularization via laser has shown clinical promise, issues remain with the use of laser energy as the means of channel formation. A summary of experimental and conceptual limitations of laser TMR is outlined in Table 5.1.

The physical creation of channels in the myocardium via laser energy involves multiple mechanistic steps. Several of these steps have significant untoward side-effects. In general, laser tissue ablation involves two linked but distinct processes: a thermal process and an acoustic process. A thermal vaporization process starts

| Table 5.1 Potential limitations of laser-mediated transmyocardial revascularization |
| --- |
| *Experimental limitations* |
| Thermal injury |
| Acoustic injury |
| Myocardial injury at a distance from the channel |
| Excessive channel (wall) fibrosis |
| Limited scar angiogenesis |
| Microbubble formation |
| Myocardial tissue fragment generation |
| Embolic risk |
| Arrhythmia risk |
| Cumbersome power source |
| Cost |
| |
| *Conceptual limitations* |
| Limited control of extent of myocardial injury |
| Unnecessary myocyte damage/dropout |
| Limited availability to vary injury variables/methods |
| Limited ability to deliver pharmacological, cellular and genetic agents for therapeutic synergy |

as photons of laser energy are absorbed by tissue water and proteins.[10] This absorption leads to a local increase in tissue temperature and pressure, followed by tissue desiccation and thermal vaporization. Some of the latent heat remains in the tissue and is transmitted to the adjacent layers to cause peri-channel thermal injury and charring.

The acoustic "pop" heard when the pulsed lasers are fired into tissue follows a cavitation phenomenon.[18] As tissue is rapidly heated, water contained within the tissue is rapidly vaporized to form bubbles of hot gases that expand at several hundred cm/s. When the flow of photons ceases, bubbles collapse and cause an audible "pop", sending acoustic shock waves through the tissue. These shock waves have the ability to stun and injure adjacent tissue layers.

Heating of the myocardium at the channel site has pathobiological consequences. Although effective in ablating a zone of tissue to form a channel, myocardial heating in the channel during channel formation creates a thermal gradient in the tissue adjacent to the channel. This peri-channel heating results in additional myocyte injury, death, and dropout. A basic tenet of direct myocardial revascularization is to create channels without excessive injury and loss of residual myocardial function. From this perspective, the added heat burden retained in the myocardium is unnecessary and may be detrimental. Recent histopathological studies of laser TMR showed that myocardial microvessels contacted by laser energy are thermally sealed and may be charred in the procedure.[19] Significant thermal myocardial injury associated with laser TMR results in increased channel-wall and myocardial fibrosis.[20] Microvessels adjacent to healed laser channels do not appear to reconnect to new capillaries associated with healing angiogenesis.[21].

Thermoacoustic energy causes additional trauma to the myocardium, beyond that confined to the immediate channel zone during channel formation. Both the holmium: YAG and $CO_2$ lasers create a rim of acoustic injury around the channel lumen that incites an inflammatory response.[22,23] Although some degree of inflammatory response may be beneficial in promoting local angiogenesis, excessive inflammation is detrimental and results in increased scar, fibrosis, and greater myocyte dropout. Acoustic shock-wave injury has also been observed to occur at a distance from the channel, in non-contiguous myocardium, with observed myocyte disarray.[24] These multiple-component injury mechanisms have the net effect of causing myocardial injury beyond that necessary for channel creation, leading to additional functional myocyte loss.

Embolic risk is increased with laser TMR. Laser-mediated acoustic shock waves impact the myocardium in a "jack hammer" fashion. As such, during the process of channel formation, many myocardial tissue fragments are ejected from the channel zone into the left ventricle.[13] In addition to tissue fragments, acoustic cavitation and heat mediated steam formation generates microbubbles.[10,25] These bubbles are shown readily by transeophageal echocardiography during laser

TMR.[8] Tissue fragments and microbubbles are a significant embolic risk to the patient and give an increased stroke risk. Grocott[13] clinically showed that cerebral embolization occurs during laser TMR, and that the quantity of emboli was significant.[13]

In terms of ergonomics, laser devices are typically cumbersome and require much maintenance and upkeep. Clinical lasers are usually large devices, making tableside positioning in the operating room or catheterization laboratory difficult. Laser TMR is also expensive for a medical centre to implement, with significant capital and per-case costs.[14,15]

## What is mechanical myocardial channeling?

In an attempt to address many of the limitations of laser TMR, an alternative mechanical means of direct myocardial revascularization has been developed. This technique is referred to as "mechanical myocardial channeling" (MMC). The basic rationale behind this approach has been to develop a physical method, readily adaptable to surgical as well as percutaneous therapeutic practice, which incorporates the essence of direct revascularization, ie, the creation of discrete myocardial channels. Although it is becoming increasingly clear that channels acutely created do not, for the most part, remain patent in the long run, creation of clean "surgical" channels may offer additional therapeutic benefit.

MMC provides the best opportunity for persistent channel or channel remnant patency. Although most TMR channels close, histopathological studies of myocardium from patients after TMR show that up to 10% of channels may remain patent. Mechanical channeling offers potential advantages here. Cleanly created channels typically heal well, with less scarring and extent of tissue damage, thus providing the best chance for long-term patency. Experimental studies have shown that mechanically created channels that do remain patent have reduced extents of wall fibrosis compared with laser, offering an advantage in terms of reduced diffusional barriers.

Most of the benefit of MMC is derived not from acute channeling but from the injury and secondary healing process that is associated with channeling. The physical process of penetration and tissue removal from the myocardium stimulates a cascade of post-injury healing responses, which lead to the net development of local islands of angiogenesis and vasculogenesis.[26] As such, channel creation (ie, induction of defined myocardial injury) without unnecessary supplemental myocardial injury and functional drop-out, is the goal of mechanical channeling. A mechanical method that uses metal cutting surfaces provides a back-to-basics approach to channel creation.

MMC achieves local channel formation via a combination of rotary coring and simultaneous vacuum tissue extraction. Rotary coring needles of adjustable

**45**

length are mechanically driven to rapidly penetrate and traverse the myocardium. Coring typically occurs at several thousand rpm. The depth of penetration may be adjusted, being full thickness for surgical (epi-endocardial) channeling, or partial for percutaneous (endo-meso) channeling. Coring needles are typically made of hard biocompatible metals with an ultra-smooth cutting edge. These ultra-sharp cutting edges pierce, separate, and extract tissue to create a clean "surgical" channel-tissue interface, without significant adjacent myocardial torsional or thermal injury.

Coring occurs simultaneously with applied channel suction, which assures rapid purchase, traversal, and retrieval of all tissue cores. Suction is cycled in the coring process, resulting in minimal ventricular blood loss. Suction during coring also aids device maintenance, keeping the coring mechanism free of clogging tissue and debris. Extracted tissue may also be retrieved and further examined with this system.

The overall process of MMC involves several steps. First, the device is positioned on the myocardium at the site of desired channel formation (Figure 5.1 a). Second, the device is stabilized to assure perpendicular penetration and absence of device movement during channeling (Figure 5.1 b). Next, the device is actuated, and the rotary coring piercing needle system traverses the myocardium (Figure 5.1 c). The needle then reverses its linear translation to backout of the myocardium (Figure 5.1 d). The device is then released from its channeling position and is ready for new channel formation.

## What devices may be used for mechanical myocardial channeling?

Two broad classes of devices have been designed for MMC: surgical or transmyocardial mechanical channeling devices (TMC); and percutaneous myocardial channeling devices (PMC).

### TMC devices

The TMC system is a mechanical instrument designed to perform myocardial revascularization via the creation of 1 mm transmural myocardial channels during cardiothoracic surgery. The current system consists of a hand-held device with an extended cannula and rotating hollow coring needle (Figure 5.2). The coring needle is connected via a cable to a console that provides the mechanism for a several-thousand-rpm rotation as well as a controlled source of vacuum. The device creates transmural channels through the left ventricular wall by mechanical coring from the epicardial surface through the myocardium into the

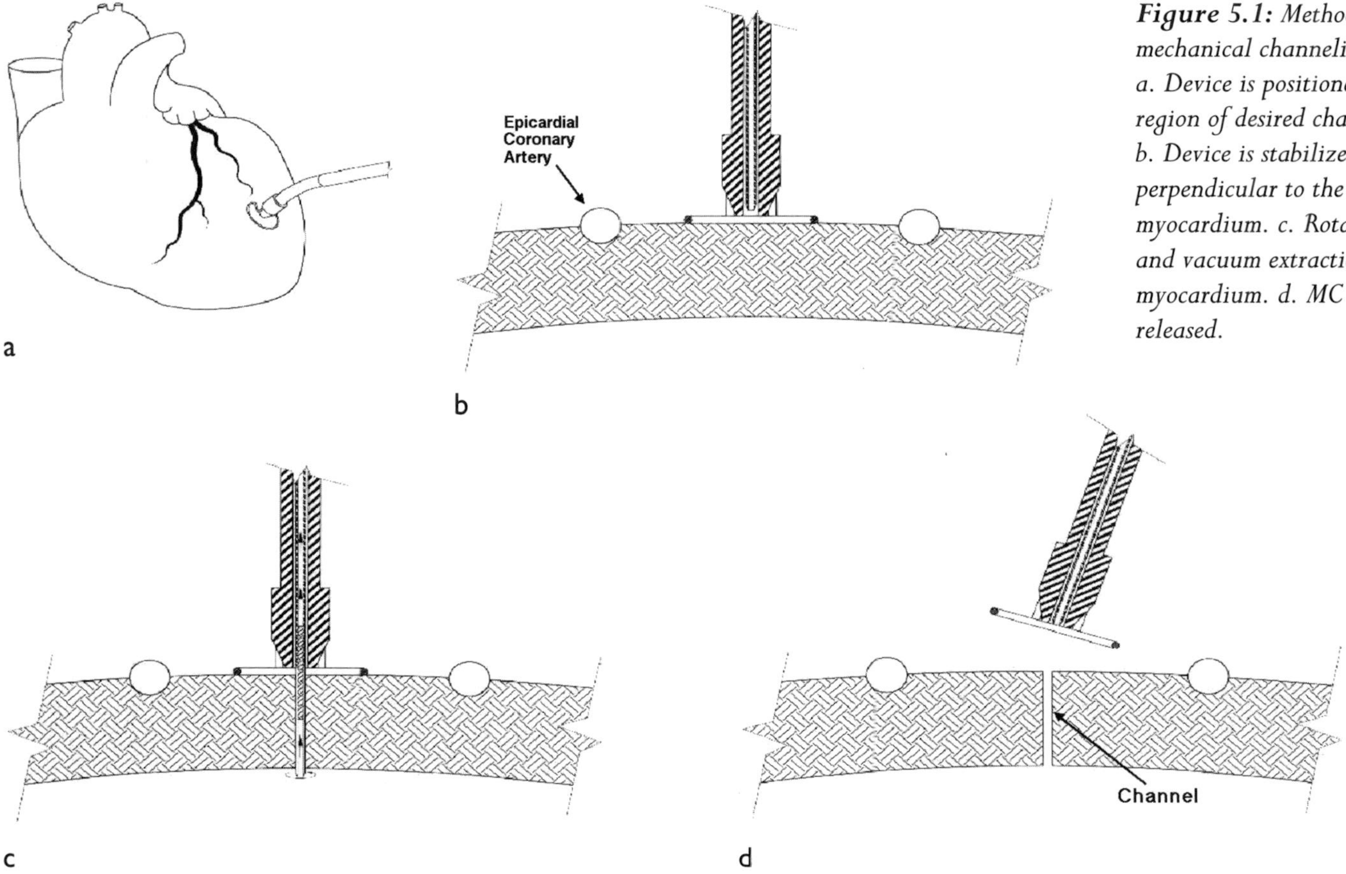

*Figure 5.1: Method of mechanical channeling. a. Device is positioned in the region of desired channeling. b. Device is stabilized perpendicular to the myocardium. c. Rotary coring and vacuum extraction of myocardium. d. MC device is released.*

Epicardial Coronary Artery

Channel

a

b

c

d

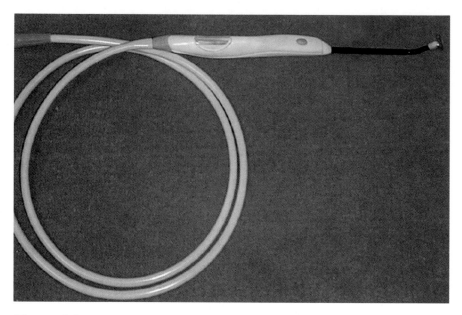

**Figure 5.2:** *Transmyocardial mechanical channeling device. Functional handle with coring needle and vacuum extraction means.*

left ventricular cavity. Tissue cores are continuously aspirated during the channeling process. The thickness of the myocardium and the distance for needle travel are determined before channeling via an external depth gauge or through use of 2D echocardiography. The channeling device is actuated via a mechanism on the device handle. A rotating hollow needle advances forward to create the channels with vacuum to aspirate the core into a vacuum container. Bleedback from the channeling process is detectable through an observation window, thereby confirming complete penetration through the myocardium. The procedure may be repeated at differing myocardial locations to generate an array of channels. The clinical version of the TMC system incorporates an adjustable articulating tip to position the TMC device on the epicardial surface of the anterior or posterior region of the heart. A stabilizer ring allows immobilization of the cannula at the surface. The needle travel distance is electronically controlled.

## PMC devices

PMC systems are catheter-based devices with a matching drive console designed to allow controlled percutaneous mechanical channeling from an intraventricular position. Devices are compatible with conventional percutaneous sheath systems

(8–9 Fr). Catheters are of a durable design, with adequate body to readily allow torque and linear movement translation. Catheters contain a means of internal mechanical coring. Coring catheters also have a mechanism for tip angulation. Catheters are designed to track within an intraventricular guide catheter, which is placed atraumatically across the aortic valve by use of a leading wire and cannula system. The combination of guide catheter and coring catheter translation, articulation, and torquing guarantees full intraventricular endocardial surface access, to allow channeling in all potential myocardial regions that may benefit from PMC.

PMC catheters are designed to stabilize against the endocardial surface once a desired location for channel formation has been selected. A rotary coring needle system, contained within the body of the catheter, may then be actuated from an external handle device to extract a channel rapidly. As opposed to the TMC device, PMC devices are specifically designed to allow for only partial thickness coring ($\leq$5 mm in depth). This feature provides safety, and prevents full thickness channel formation and perforation.

The proposed indication for use of TMC and PMC systems is the treatment of debilitating angina and regional ischemia associated with advanced or extensive coronary artery disease, which would be otherwise poorly or incompletely treated by conventional approaches. Channeling is intended for the treatment of viable regions of the left ventricle where location, extent, and severity of coronary disease precludes effective treatment with conventional revascularization (CABG, PTCA).

## How does MMC simplify direct revascularization and overcome the limitations of laser TMR?

MMC simplifies direct revascularization by providing an easier, less technologically cumbersome means for myocardial channel formation. MMC surgical and percutaneous systems, as described above, are easy to set up, and use mobile devices for channel creation. Further, these systems allow control and modulation of several injury variables associated with channel formation. Techniques can be improved as the science and biology of direct myocardial revascularization evolves and is increasingly understood over time. MMC also provides the opportunity to enhance direct revascularization in that the method and devices, being modular, allow for the addition of potentially synergistic pharmacological and cellular therapies for enhanced therapeutic outcome.

On a practical level, MMC forms channels via a simple reliable energy form and device means. TMC and PMC use mechanical kinetic energy to induce torsional and shearing forces, thereby physically cutting myocardial tissue. This mechanism of tissue excision uses the same energy form and principle as surgical

**49**

cutting. The biological response to tissue cutting via knife shearing is well understood and may be well controlled. Mechanical channel formation, via coring needles with sharp cutting surfaces, does not impart the degree of tissue heating, either intra- or peri-channel, as occurs with lasers. Further, mechanical cutting does not have associated acoustic shock injury. Elimination of myocardial shock waves further reduces local as well as distant myocardial injury. Whittaker and colleagues[27] in experimental studies in the rat directly compared the healing response in mechanical versus laser channel formation. They observed that laser-made channels were associated with significantly more channel-associated fibrosis than mechanical needle-made channels (mean width of fibrosis 430 $\pm$ 50 $\mu$ versus 180 $\pm$ 30 $\mu$, p < 0.001). In subsequent ischemic challenge studies, needle-made channels gave greater myocardial protection than laser-made channels. The researchers proposed that needle-created channels provide more protection owing to reduced damage to the surrounding tissue than the relatively extensive damage observed with the holmium: YAG laser.

The demonstration of less myocardial scarring, fibrosis, and channel remnant wall fibrosis thickness with mechanical channeling versus laser offers several potential advantages. For remnant channels that do remain patent and/or communicating with myocardial capillaries and sinusoids, the presence of a thinner layer of fibrosis offers potential benefit. Thinner layers of fibrosis reduce the diffusional barrier in the circulatory path. This allows more oxygen, nutrient, and macromolecule exchange than may occur in the presence of a collagenous barrier. Further, having more extensive regions of collagenous scar form, rather than small regions of transitional matrix, provides a less favourable milieu for angiogenesis and capillary sprouting.

Mechanical channel formation also provides an added device safety. The acoustic impact of laser channel formation imparts compressive expulsive forces, with vectors directly aimed at the ventricular cavity. As channels are formed, microbubbles and tissue fragments may be detected entering the left ventricle (LV).[8] By contrast, the risk of emboli, either microbubble or tissue debris, is significantly lessened with mechanical channeling. The mechanism of coring, as discussed above, with knife-edge tissue cutting, shearing, and continuous vacuum extraction, does not impart any expulsive or ejecting forces to the ventricular cavity. This, coupled with continuous suction, favours tissue movement directly away from the LV, and eliminates the possibility of tissue remnants entering the ventricle and systemically embolizing.

MMC also has reduced arrhythmia risk. Laser TMR has been observed clinically to induce significant ventricular irritability with resultant PVCs and burst of ventricular tachycardia. For these reasons, pulsed laser TMR systems have to be synchronized with the ECG. Needle puncture of the myocardium, by contrast, does not induce the same degree of ventricular irritability. Several early studies have in fact assessed the use of myocardial needle puncture as an actual means of reducing ventricular arrhythmias.[4]

On an ergonomic level, mechanical channel formation may be accomplished with greater reliability and reduced maintenance compared with lasers. As described above, mechanical channeling devices may be powered via small drive units free from significant upkeep. Small power units may be mounted on a mobile tripod, or placed on or adjacent to the catheterization table. Mechanical drive systems remove the need for heavy gauge power cords, cooling mechanisms, and significant power requirements typically associated with laser devices, thereby making the operative or interventional workfield less cluttered. These simpler devices may be made at much lower cost than lasers. As such, lower costs will limit the effect on the health-care dollar, making mechanical channeling therapy more widely available to patients in need.

In addition to the above potential advantages of mechanical channeling, this technique also addresses several conceptual limitations of laser TMR. Channel making via laser, as outlined above, comprises multiple mechanisms and imparts several forms of injury to the myocardium. As such, laser energy, even if pulsed or altered in terms of fluence, sequence, and duration of application, still affords limited means for controlling the extent of injury and the relative contribution of different component mechanisms. Mechanical coring, by contrast, may achieve channeling with greater injury control. As our understanding evolves of the relative contribution of components of injury to the overall late healing and angiogenic response of the myocardium, mechanical channeling will readily allow modification of the mode and extent of tissue injury. As such, mechanical channeling may be viewed as a modular platform for physical manipulation of the myocardium at the time of channel formation.

Mechanical channeling can also readily deliver additional therapeutic agents to the myocardium, Significant investigation is underway in the use of growth factors, either as genes or actual protein, for enhanced regional angiogenesis.[28] TMC and PMC devices will allow direct injection or deposition of many potential therapeutics including pharmacological, cellular, and genetic therapies. Mechanical myocardial penetration will readily allow such deposition contemporaneous to or immediately after channeling. The advantage of mechanical channeling devices is that they provide a means of direct myocardial injection, coordinated with a means of myocardial injury, which minimally inactivates the adjunctive biotherapeutic. There is no risk of thermal inactivation or denaturation of a growth factor with cool needle injection. By contrast, laser energy will readily inactivate and denature bioactive compounds, either directly exposed to energy or secondarily altered by local heating.

## What are the acute whole animal and myocardial responses to MMC?

Many studies have been done to date to assess the acute whole animal and myocardial effects of mechanical channeling. Results of these studies are summarized below.

Mechanical channeling has been done to date in more than 60 pigs using the surgical TMC device described above. Myocardial access using thoracotomy and median sternotomy has been done. All regions of the left ventricle have been readily accessed with the TMC device. Mechanical channeling has been done on the anterior, lateral, and posterior walls of the porcine left ventricle. 30 channels, on average, have been placed per heart. To date there have been no intra- or peri-procedural deaths associated with TMC. An example of a series of channels placed in an array on the porcine anterior wall may be seen below (Figure 5.3 a). The transmural nature of these channels may be seen in the accompanying photomicrograph (Figure 5.3 b).

a                      b

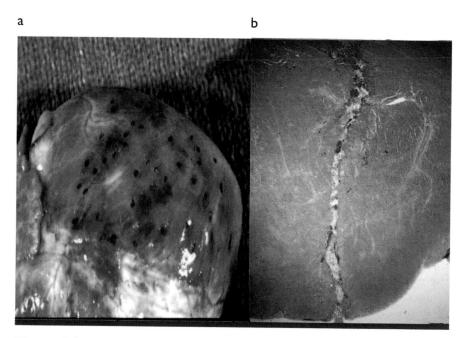

**Figure 5.3:** *a. Anterior wall of pig heart with array of mechanically placed channels. b. Photomicrograph of acutely placed channel. Note transmural extension.*

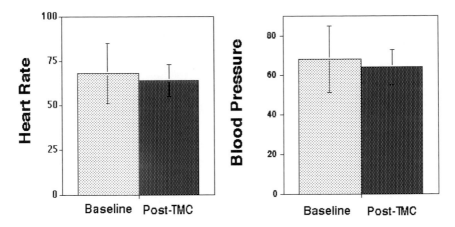

*Figure 5.4:* Hemodynamic response to TMC. Heart rate (left panel) and blood pressure (right panel) did not vary.

TMC has generally been well tolerated in the pigs studied. Heart rate and blood pressure have varied little, comparing baseline with post-procedure. In a recently reported acute study[16] heart rates were 124 ± 20 pre-procedure versus 137 ± 9 post-TMC (p = 0.16). Similarly, blood pressure was 68 ± 17 versus 64 ± 9 post-TMC (p = 0.6, Figure 5.4).

Mechanical channeling has not resulted in significant myocardial ischemia. In a study of seven normal pigs, after placement of 30 channels in the anterior wall mean ST segment elevation in leads $V_4 - V_6$ was less than 1 mm (0 mm at baseline *vs* 0.43 + 1.05 mm post TMC, p = 0.3).[16] This slight ST deviation was typically transient, reverting to pre-TMC baseline shortly after the procedure.

MMC was not associated with significant arrhythmia generation. During the process of channeling an occasional PVC or couplet was detected. No episodes of sustained or non-sustained ventricular tachycardia or ventricular fibrillation occurred during or in the post-procedural recovery period of TMC. No supraventricular arrhythmias occurred.

Mechanical channeling was well tolerated by the left ventricle in terms of ventricular function. Two dimensional echocardiography was done on pigs before and immediately after TMC. Using the AHA/ACC scoring system (1 = normal, 2 = hypokinetic, 3 = akinetic, 4 = dykinetic, 5 = aneurysmal), in several studies post-TMC wall motion scores did not vary from baseline (1 baseline *vs* 1 post-TMC).[17]

# What are the chronic myocardial healing responses to TMC?

The overall goal of both laser TMR and MMC is to alter the myocardial substrate to reduce its ischemic potential. Many mechanisms have been postulated to underlie the chronic efficacy of direct revascularization, including persistent channel patency, secondary angiogenesis, and regional denervation, but current thinking supports induction of angiogenesis as the predominant mechanism providing therapeutic benefit. As such, a goal for mechanical channeling has been to induce secondary healing-associated angiogenesis, while limiting the extent of excessive myocardial injury.

Studies have been done to assess the histopathological response of the myocardium to TMC. TMC was done on the anterior wall of 18 normal pigs. At 60 days after healing myocardium was subjected to gross and histopathological analysis.

## Gross pathology after 60-day healing

In all hearts, the left ventricular anterior wall was intact, without evidence of shape alteration, bulging, or aneurysm formation. No evidence of gross anterior wall scarring, fibrosis, or thinning was observed. Localized regions of epicardial to pericardial adhesion formation were detected, with focal minimal fibrin deposition. Neither pericardial nor epicardial thrombus was observed.

## Histopathology after 60-day healing

Channel remnants were detectable in transmural sections of the anterior wall. Of 20 channels examined, all were found fully healed and filled with proteoglycan-collagenous matrix that contained multiple types and sizes of vessels. Typically, remnants were consistent with scar at various stages of maturity. Channel tracts clearly stained positive for collagen with trichrome staining. An example of a healed channel remnant is shown below (Figure 5.5). Channel remnants averaged 1135 ± 165 microns. Adjacent myocardium, both immediate to the channel border and several mm from the channel, appeared histologically intact and healthy. No evidence of significant myocyte drop-out, fibrosis, or inflammatory infiltrate was observed. Unlike laser channeling, TMC did not produce charring of the channels nor did it coagulate the adjacent myocardial tissue.

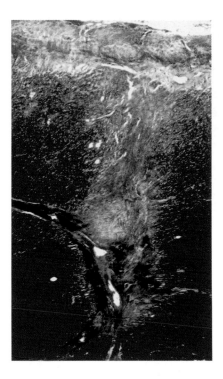

**Figure 5.5:** *Cross-section of myocardium 60 days after TMC. Note channel remnant filled with collagenous material.*

## Channel angiogenesis and vasculogenesis

Significant vascularity in the region of the channel remnant and in the per-channel myocardium was noted in the histological analysis. A wide mixture of vessel types was detected (Figure 5.6). Capillaries (< 25 μ, Figure 5.7), small arterioles (25–200 μ) and medium sized arterioles (200–400 μ, Figure 5.8) were seen within and immediately adjacent to the healed channel. An increase in capillary density (20.1 ± 9.6/25× field), small arteriole density (5.3 ± 2.5/10× field), and medium arteriole density (0.76 ± 0.23/10× field) compared with normal myocardium was noted within the region of the healed channel remnant. The increase in capillary density observed provides direct evidence for post-TMC healing angiogenesis. Interestingly, the increase in small and medium sized arteriolar density shows coordinate "vasculogenesis". This increase in arteriolar structures appears to date to be a unique finding of mechanical TMC. While the mechanisms underlying this increase in larger arterial conduits with TMC is incompletely understood, the finding of vessel structures with greater cross-sectional areas than capillaries is particularly intriguing. Larger muscular arteries

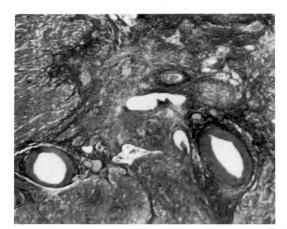

**Figure 5.6:** *Mixed vascularity of channel remnant. Note presence of capillaries and multi-layered vessels (small arterioles).*

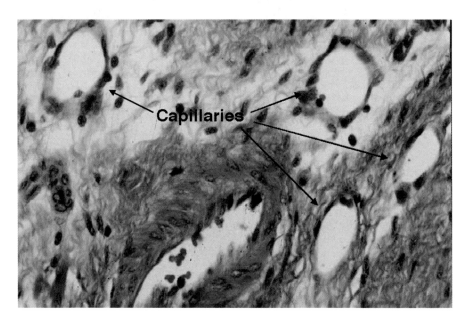

**Figure 5.7:** *Capillaries typically seen within channel remnant. Note wide distribution of sizes.*

are of greater physiological relevance for reducing ischemia, since vessels with larger cross-sectional area are better suited for provision of bulk blood flow to the ischemic myocardium than small capillaries.

**56**

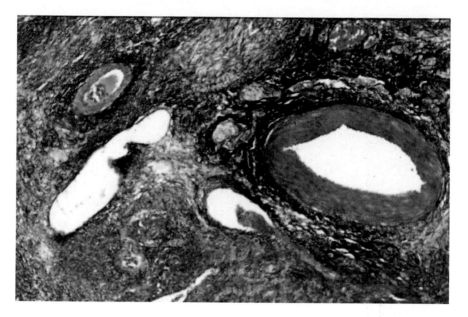

**Figure 5.8:** *Small and medium sized arterioles in healed TMC zone. The appearance of a "vasculogenic" response is best to provide adequate cross-section for blood flow.*

## Does the strategy of "TMC + healing" limit ischemic consequences of acute coronary occlusion?

The ultimate goal of mechanical channeling is to provide enhanced myocardial protection in the face of ischemia. As such, experiments have recently been done to assess the ability of the strategy of "TMC followed by a period of 60-day healing" to provide myocardial protection in acute ischemia. Based on the above findings of significant neovascularization accompanying TMC healing, it was thought that the post-TMC healing process and other secondary beneficial healing responses may alter the myocardium, allowing it to better handle an acute ischemic insult compared with sham controls.

A stringent experimental preparation was used to test this hypothesis. Normal pigs underwent TMC of the anterior wall from the level of the second diagonal to the apex. An average of 30 channels was placed on the anterior wall. Pigs were allowed to heal. Sham controls were generated, treated identically but without channeling. At 60 days post-intervention all pigs were subjected to acute

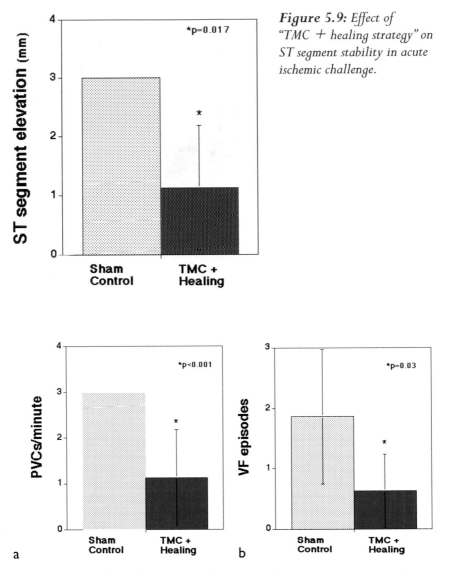

*Figure 5.9:* Effect of "TMC + healing strategy" on ST segment stability in acute ischemic challenge.

*Figure 5.10:* Effect of "TMC + healing strategy" on ventricular ectopy (a) and ventricular fibrillation (b) in acute ischemic challenge.

ischemic challenge, in the form of acute occlusion of the LAD between the first and second diagonal. The results of this study are summarized below.

Ischemia was monitored via examination of ST segment deviation from baseline. After 60 min of LAD occlusion, ST segment elevation in leads $V_4 - V_6$ was significantly less in pigs conditioned via TMC + healing than in the sham conditioned controls ($1.8 + 2.6$ mm *vs* $5.9 + 2.0$ mm, $p = 0.017$, Figure 5.9). Similarly, the frequency of premature ventricular ectopy ($1.13 \pm 1.05$ PVCs/min *vs* $3.0 \pm 0$ [sham control], $p < 0.001$, Figure 5.10 a) and the incidence of ventricular fibrillation episodes ($0.63 \pm 0.7$ *vs* $1.86 \pm 1.12$ [sham control], $p = 0.03$, Figure 5.10 b) were reduced as well by TMC conditioning. These findings suggest that the process of TMC and subsequent myocardial healing protects against acute ischemic challenge. Although many protective mechanisms may underlie this protective effect, these observations coupled with the finding of increased vascular density in healed channel remnants suggest that a neovascularization mechanism predominates in the observed ischemic protection.

## How might MMC be combined with pharmacological and biological therapies for enhanced angiogenesis and vasculogenesis?

A potential advantage of MMC versus other means of direct myocardial revascularization stems from its ability to deliver supplemental therapeutics locally. Direct myocardial access, either via epicardial or endocardial approaches, coupled with the coordinate ability to contemporaneously deliver agents at the time of channeling, underlies this potential therapeutic synergy. As discussed above, TMC provides penetrating myocardial access and allows agent delivery via methods that will not significantly denature adjunctive therapeutic agents.

Mechanical needle puncture of the myocardium may be readily coordinated with delivery of a wide variety of synergistic therapeutics. Agents for potential consideration include various growth factors such as basic fibroblast growth factor (bFGF),[29] vascular endothelial growth factor (VEGF),[30] platelet derived endothelial growth factor (PDECG),[31] transforming growth factor-$\beta$ (TGF-$\beta$),[32] tumour necrosis factor-$\alpha$ (TNF-$\alpha$,[33] interleukin-1,[34] interleukin-8,[35] and leptin.[36] Mechanical channeling devices may also directly deliver genes for angiogenic substances, either as naked DNA (eg, cDNA for phVEGF$_{121}$)[37] or as transfection viral vectors (eg, adenovirus encoding VEGF$_{121}$).[38] Further, mechanical channeling devices may also be used to deliver precursor endothelial cells or mature endothelial cells directly into ischemic zones.[39]

## Summary and conclusions

MMC is a simple, readily performed technique for direct revascularization of the myocardium. Devices for mechanical channeling, whether surgical or percutaneous, use mechanical energy for tissue extraction and removal. These

**59**

devices are inherently simpler, more ergonomic, easier to maintain, and less expensive than laser TMR systems. The mechanical channeling technique effectively creates clean-cut reproducible myocardial channels without significant whole animal or myocardial effects. This mode of channel creation effectively creates channels without the induction of potentially unnecessary "bystander" myocardial injury. In multiple studies in the pig model, TMC was free of acute procedural deaths and did not induce significant ischemia, arrhythmias, or regional wall motion abnormalities. Chronically, hearts treated with TMC heal with channel involution and scarring. Interestingly, channel remnants are highly vascular, with a significant increase in capillary, small, and medium arteriolar density. This increase in arterioles (or "vasculogenic" response) is ideal since it affords increased blood perfusion potential over simple angiogenesis. Hearts conditioned by the process of TMC plus healing appear to be more resilient to acute ischemic challenge, with reduced signs of ischemia, electrical, and mechanical instability. A true advantage of MMC is its modular design and synergistic capability with pharmacotherapy. While effective in its own right, MMC may potentially be combined with bioactive therapeutics for treatment synergy. MMC, in its initial form as described above, must be viewed as a first step toward simpler yet more effective means of direct myocardial revascularization. Through continued coordinate advances in device engineering, cell biology, pharmacology, and genetic engineering, enhanced synergistic devices and methods may lead to long-term highly effective myocardial revascularization.

## Acknowledgment

This work was supported by an educational grant from Angiotrax, Inc., Sunnyvale, CA, USA.

## References

1. Sen PK, Udwadia TE, Kinare SG, Parulkar GB. Transmyocardial acupuncture. *J Thorac Cardiovasc Surg* 1965; **50**: 181–9.

2. Goldman A, Greenstone Presuss FS, Strauss SH, Chang ES. Experimental methods for producing a collateral circulation to the heart directly from the left ventricle. *J Thorac Surg* 1956; **6**: 163–71.

3. Khazei AH, Kime WP, Papadopolous C, Cowley RA. Myocardial canalization: a new method of myocardial revascularization. *Ann Thorac Surg* 1968; **6**: 163–71.

4. White M, Hershey JE. Multiple transmyocardial puncture revascularization in

refractory ventricular fibrillation due to myocardial ischemia. *Ann Thorac Surg* 1968; **168:** 871–5.

5.   Mirhoseini M, Cayton MM. Revascularization of the heart by laser. *J Microsurg* 1981; **2:** 253–60.

6.   Mirhoseini M, Shelgikar S, Cayton MM. New concepts of revascularization of the myocardium. *Ann Thorac Surg* 1988; **45:** 415–20.

7.   Cooley DA, Frazier OH, Kadipasaoglu KA, Lindenmeir MH, Pehlivanoglu S, Kolff JW. Transmyocardial laser revascularization: clinical experience with twelve months follow-up. *J Thorac Cardiovasc Surg* 1996; **111:** 791–7.

8.   Horvath KA, Manning F, Cummings N, Sherman SK, Cohn L. Transmyocardial laser revascularization: operative techniques and clinical results at two years. *J Thorac Cardiovasc Surg* 1996; **111:** 1047–53.

9.   Horvath KA, Cohn LH, Cooley DA et al. Transmyocardial laser revascularization: results of a multi-center trial using TLR as a sole therapy for end-stage coronary artery disease. *J Thorac Cardiovasc Surg* 1997; **113:** 645–53.

10.  Jansen ED, Frenz M, Kadipasaoglu KA et al. Laser-tissue interaction during transmyocardial revascularization. *Ann Thorac Surg* 1997; **63:** 640–7.

11.  Hartman RA, Whittaker P. The physics of transmyocardial laser revascularization. *J Clin Laser Med Surg* 1997; **15:** 255–9.

12.  Jaques SL. Laser-tissue interactions: photochemical, photothermal and mechanical. *Surg Clin North Am* 1992; **72:** 531–8.

13.  Grocott HP, Amory DW, Lowry E, Newman MF, Lowe JE, Clements FM. Cerebral embolization during transmyocardial laser revascularization. *J Thorac Cardiovasc Surg* 1997; **114:** 856–8.

14.  Kruger K. TMR Report 1996–1997. Montgomery Securities, San Francisco, CA: 49.

15.  Lemaitre D, Cohen M. 5th Annual cardiology device update. SG Cowen, New York, NY, 1999: 162.

16.  Slepian MJ, LePrince PN, Toporoff B et al. Transmyocardial channelling: a mechanical alternative to laser transmyocardial revascularization. *Am J Cardiol* 1998; **82** (suppl 7A): 17S.

17.  Slepian MJ, LePrince PN, Toporoff B et al. Acute mechanical transmyocardial channeling provides myocardial protection for ischemia. *J Am Coll Cardiol* 1999; **33:** 341A.

18.  Muller GJ, Dorschel K, Schladach B. Transmyocardial laser revascularization: a matter of right wavelength. In: *TMLR: Management of Coronary Artery Disease*. Klein M, Schulte HD, Gams E (eds). Springer, Berlin, 1998; 123–9.

19.  Sigel JE, Abramovich CM, Lytle BW, Ratcliff NB. Transmyocardial laser

**61**

revascularization: three sequential autopsy cases. *J Thorac Cardiovasc Surg* 1998; **115:** 1381–5.

20.  Nath S, Haines DE. Biophysics and pathology of catheter energy delivery systems. *Prog Cardiovasc Dis* 1995; **37:** 185–204.

21.  R Virami. Personal communication, 1999.

22.  Zheng S, Kloner RA, Whittaker P. Ablation and coagulation of myocardial tissue by means of a pulsed holmium: YAG laser. *Am Heart J* 1993; **126:** 1471–7.

23.  Kohmoto T, DeRosa CM, Yamamoto N et al. Evidence of vascular growth associated with laser treatment of normal canine myocardium. *Ann Thorac Surg* 1998; **65:** 1360–7.

24.  Fisher PE, Khomoto T, DeRosa CM, Spotnitz HM, Smith CR, Burkhoff D. Histologic analysis of transmyocardial channels: comparison of CO2 and holmium : YAG lasers. *Ann Thorac Surg* 1997; **64:** 466–72.

25.  Van Erven L, van Leeuwen TG, Post MJ, van der Veen MJ, Velema E, Borst C. Mid-infrared laser ablation of the arterial wall: mechanical origin of "acoustic" wall damage and its effect on wall healing. *J Thorac Cardiovasc Surg* 1992; **104:** 1053–9.

26.  Slepian MJ. Unpublished observation, 1999.

27.  Whittaker P, Rakusan K, Kloner RA. Transmural channels can protect ischemic tissue: assessment of long-term myocardial response to laser- and needle-made channels. *Circulation* 1996; **93:** 143–52.

28.  Rivard A, Isner JM. Angiogenesis and vasculogenesis in treatment of cardiovascular disease. *Mol Med* 1998; **4:** 429–40.

29.  Baffour R, Berman J, Garb JL, Rhee SW, Kaufman J, Friedmann P. Enhanced angiogenesis and growth of collaterals by in vivo administration of recombinant basic fibroblast growth factor in a rabbit model of acute lower limb ischemia: dose-response effect of basic fibroblast growth factor. *J Vasc Surg* 1992; **16:** 181–91.

30.  Takeshita S, Zheng LP, Brogi E et al. Therapeutic angiogenesis: a single intra-arterial bolus of vascular endothelial growth factor augments revascularization in a rabbit ischemic hindlimb model. *J Clin Invest* 1994; **93:** 662–70.

31.  Ishikawa F, Miyazono K, Hellman U et al. Identification and angiogeneic activity and the cloning and expression of platelet-derived endothelial cell growth factor. *Nature* 1998; **338:** 557–62.

32.  Chang HL, Gillet N, Figari I, Lopez AR, Palladino MA, Derynck R. Increased transforming growth factor $\beta$ expression inhibits cell proliferation in vitro yet increases tumorigenicity and tumor growth of meth A sarcoma cells. *Cancer Res* 1993; **53:** 4391–8.

33.  Frater-Schroeder MF, Risau W, Hallmann R, Gautschi P, Bohlem P. Tumor

necrosis factor-a, a potent inhibitor of endothelial cell growth in vitro, is angiogenic in vivo. *Proc Nat Acad Sci USA* 1987; **84:** 5277–81.

34. Montesano RL, Orci L, Vassali P. Human endothelial cell cultures: phenotypic modulation by interleukins. *J Cell Biol* 1995; **122:** 424–34.

35. Strieter RM, Kunkel SL, Elner VM et al. Interleukin-8, a corenal factor that induces neovascularization. *Am J Pathol* 1992; **141:** 1279–84.

36. Sierra-Honigmann MR, Nath AK, Murakami C et al. Biological action of leptin as an angiogenic factor. *Science* 1998; **281:** 1683–6.

37. Takeshita S, Tsurumi Y, Couffinahl T et al. Gene transfer of naked DNA encoding for three isoforms of vascular endothelial growth factor stimulates collateral development in vivo. *Lab Invest* 1996; **75:** 487–502.

38. Mack CA, Patel SR, Schwartz EA et al. Biologic bypass with the use of adenovirus-mediated gene transfer of the complementary deoxyribonucleic acid for vascular endothelial growth factor 121 improves myocardial perfusion and function in the ischemic porcine heart. *J Thorac Cardiovasc Surg* 1998; **115:** 168–76.

39. Asahara T, Murohara T, Sullivan A et al. Isolation of putative progenitor endothelial cells for angiogenesis. *Science* 1997; **275:** 964–7.

# 6. BIOSENSE™ GUIDED DIRECT MYOCARDIAL REVASCULARIZATION

Ran Kornowski, Shmuel Fuchs and Martin B Leon

## Introduction

The Biosense™ left ventricular mapping system has been derived from a new diagnostic and navigational guidance tool that uses an ultralow magnetic-field energy source and sensor-tipped catheter electrodes to locate the exact catheter position in three-dimensional (3D) space.[1-8] The system reconstructs electromechanical maps of the left ventricle without x-ray fluoroscopy. Compared with standard fluoroscopic techniques, the Biosense™ system gives reduction in fluoroscopy exposure time, more accurate detection of arrhythmic foci and subsequent guidance for ablation treatment, and reassessment of the therapy.[9-11] In addition, this system has been used for on-line diagnosis of myocardial viability in the catheterization laboratory and for investigational protocols of percutaneous direct myocardial revascularization procedures.[6,8] The 3D electromechanical maps generated by the system are used to identify precisely viable target zones based on integration of endocardial electrical and mechanical signals. The Biosense system can be integrated with a Holmium (Ho):YAG laser for transmyocardial revascularization procedures at precise locations within the left ventricle.[12] Also, this platform technology may be used to apply intramyocardial pharmacotherapy, by injecting recombinant genes or growth factors directly into the ischemic myocardium.[13] Thus, the endomyocardial mapping and guidance system integrates in one device the identification of target zones (by electromechanical maps), catheter guidance (by location sensors), and intramyocardial therapeutics (by laser energy, local pharmacotherapy, or both) to achieve "optimal" procedural safety and efficacy with minimal x-ray radiation exposure.

## Guidance for direct myocardial revascularization

Direct myocardial revascularization (DMR) is an investigational therapeutic strategy designed to reduce anginal symptoms by use of a laser energy source or pharmacological agents (eg, angiogenic growth factors) applied directly into the ischemic myocardium. DMR can be done by either surgical or catheter-based approaches. Preliminary surgical DMR clinical trials have suggested significant reduction in angina severity, improved quality of life, and some evidence of improved myocardial perfusion in refractory coronary ischemic syndromes.[14] The catheter-based approach for DMR may be as effective as surgical DMR without the need for a thoracotomy or general anaesthesia. In addition, the catheter-based approach enables access to areas not approachable in surgical DMR (eg, the ventricular septum, the posterior wall), and allows multiple treatment sessions via a less invasive approach. Guidance for catheter-based DMR is required to: achieve optimal laser-tissue contact at treatment zones; to avoid repetitive same-site laser firing that may increase the risk of perforation; to help identify target treatment zones; and to assist with catheter navigation to the designated endomyocardial surface. Conventional navigational methods, such as bi-plane fluoroscopy and echocardiography, are limited by their two-dimensional representation, non-optimal resolution at the catheter tip–endocardial interface, inability to identify target viable treatment zones on-line, and inability to identify in advance "same site" laser firing that may contribute to myocardial perforation.

The Biosense navigational platform has been designed for catheter guidance during percutaneous DMR (Figure 6.1). The electromechanical maps are used to identify viable target zones for DMR based on intracardiac electrical and mechanical signals.[6–8] This catheter system is integrated with a laser to carry out the DMR procedure at precise locations within the left ventricle. The distal catheter-tip location and orientation are detected in real time to achieve optimal laser-tissue contact and guidance for viable treatment sites (eg, ischemic or hibernating myocardium). The exact channel location is shown in real time on the electromechanical map, and local electrical signals are traced to: minimize catheter-tip trauma (ST segment elevation); assure tip stability during laser firing; synchronize the time of laser firing with stable electrogram signals; and record the intracardiac "electrical signature" of each laser channel. Thus, the endocardial mapping and guidance concept for DMR integrates in one device the identification of target zones (by electromechanical maps), catheter guidance (by location sensors), and ablative energy (by laser system), to achieve "optimal" procedural safety and efficacy with minimal x-ray radiation exposure.

## *Biosense-DMR™ — device description*

The DMR procedure consists of left ventricular electromechanical mapping followed by endocardial laser therapy. The mapping procedure uses the following components: a triangular location pad with 3 coils generating an ultralow magnetic field energy; a stationary reference catheter with a miniature magnetic field sensor; a navigation mapping catheter with a miniature magnetic field sensor (7 Fr with deflectable tip and electrodes to give unipolar and bipolar endocardial

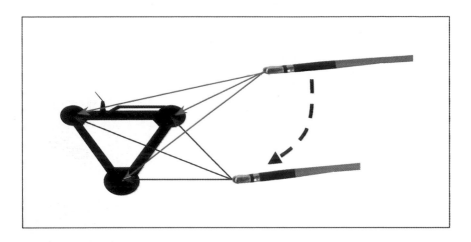

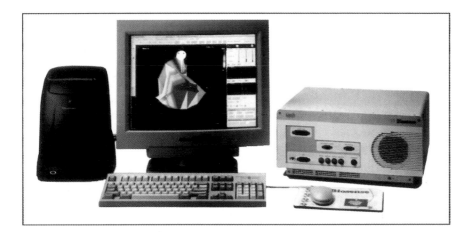

*Figure 6.1:* *The Biosense system uses low-intensity magnetic-field emittors and sensor-tipped electrodes to locate precisely the catheter position in 3D space (upper panel). A Silicon-Graphics screen and a processing unit (NOGA) are located in a workstation to show the mapping data on-line (lower panel).*

signals); and a workstation to process the information obtained from the mapping catheter and construct 3D left ventricular geometry (Figures 6.1 and 6.2). After left ventricular mapping, which can provide data on endocardial unipolar and bipolar voltage and mechanical information, a modified mapping catheter (8 Fr distal tip with a 300 μm laser fiber throughout its shaft) is exchanged for endocardial channel creation with Holmium (Ho):yttrium-aluminium-garnet

**67**

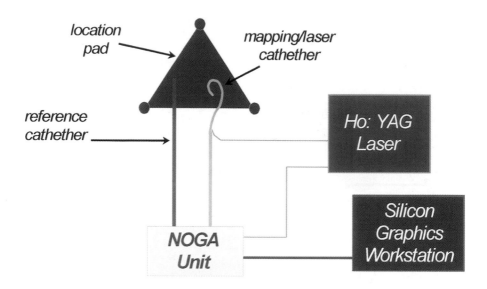

***Figure 6.2:*** *Schematic of the integrated Biosense DMR navigational and Holmium:YAG laser system: the location pad to generate electromagnetic fields, reference and mapping / lasing catheters, electromechanical mapping processing unit (NOGA) and Silicon-Graphics workstation for interpretation of the electromechanical data, and a Holmium:YAG laser system.*

(YAG) laser (Sharplan™ 2040 Ho:YAG Laser System, Allendale, NJ, USA, Figure 6.3). The Ho:YAG (@2.1 microns) has a pulse width of 250 µs and the pulse energy is set at 2 J for a single pulse per created channel. These laser energy parameters were chosen to minimize tissue damage, with less concern for channel formation and greater emphasis on triggering endogenous tissue responses in the least destructive, safest, and most reproducible way possible.[15,16] The aiming beam is 3 Mw diode laser (red), and the beam delivery is through a low OH silica optical fiber. The laser fiber has a 300 µm core diameter and is extended to the catheter tip, to maintain fiber-tissue contact, thereby reducing exposure to blood interfaces and minimizing convective energy losses. Myocardial channels are formed by placing the catheter tip on pre-defined endocardial sites *without advancing the catheter or fiber into the myocardium*. The laser is synchronized to the QRS electrocardiogram signal to operate precisely after the QRS complex.

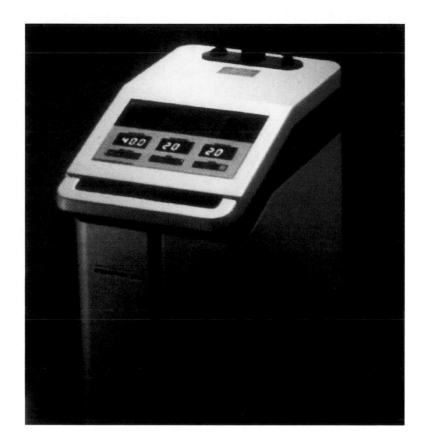

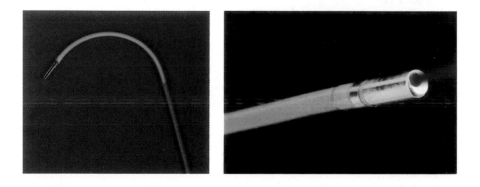

**Figure 6.3:** *(a) Sharplan Holmium:YAG laser unit. (b) Electromechanical mapping catheter containing the location sensor and tip-electrodes, integrated with a laser fiber for the left ventricular mapped direct myocardial revascularization (DMR) procedure.*

**69**

# Safety and feasibility studies in animal models

Using the Biosense™ system, 20 pigs underwent left ventricular mapping followed by percutaneous DMR with a Ho:YAG laser at 2 J × 1 pulse. Animals were sacrificed acutely at 24 h and at 3 weeks after the DMR procedure.[12] The hearts were examined grossly and microscopically, and serial CK-MB was measured up to 24 h. Sites for laser treatment were localized by binocular zoom microscope used in conjunction with the LV maps (Figure 6.4). There were no procedural complications. Animals received 13 (±2) channels in 19 (±7) min. The catheter was able to treat all regions, including the septum. There was no CK-MB elevation up to 24 h. One animal died within 1 h of the procedure. There was one sealed perforation into the subepicardial fat due to same-site laser activation. Histological assessment in the acute and 24-h groups revealed laser channels which were 3.6 (±2.2) mm long, 1.5 (±0.7) mm wide, with an entry angle of 73 ± 12° (Figure 6.5). Channels were filled with platelet thrombi acutely, and were surrounded by well-defined rims of thermal-coagulation and an "impact" zone of viable myocardium. At 3 weeks, no channels remained patent and were replaced by well-healed granulation tissue admixed with fibroblasts,

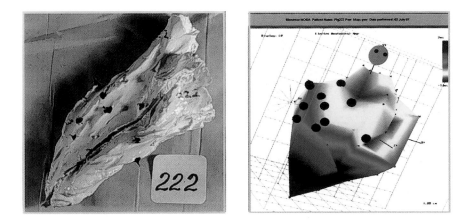

**Figure 6.4:** *Example of identification of laser-treated sites based on comparison of the NOGA electro-anatomical map with a silicon cast of the left ventricular cavity. The laser points indicated in the map (brown dots, left) correspond to the cast specimen (brown dots, right) where histological preparation was undertaken for tissue examination.*

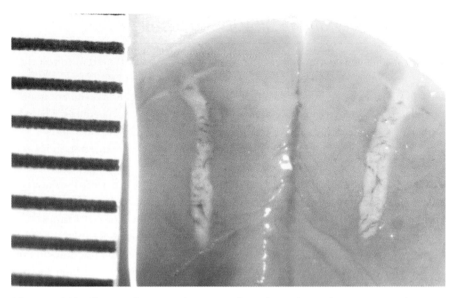

***Figure 6.5:*** *Close up horizontal section of two laser channels in a porcine heart seen under binocular power microscope (×10). Note the irregular channel borders and the thermal-injury zone ("white zone") surrounding the channel, which are typical for Ho:YAG laser-tissue effects. Channel length is about 4 mm.*

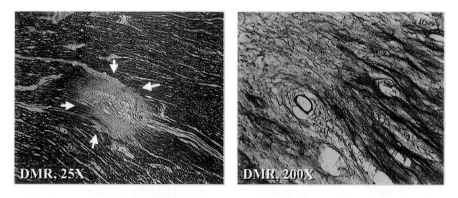

***Figure 6.6:*** *Histology taken from a healed channel site (H&E) at 4 weeks, showing granulation tissue admixed with fibroblasts and increased small-sized blood vessels in the spaces of the prior channel surrouonding.*

inflammatory cells, and small-sized vessels (Figure 6.6). This study has established the pre-clinical safety and feasibility of the percutaneous Biosense™ DMR approach and has led to a series of clinical investigations.

# Clinical safety and feasibility studies

Clinical studies are now underway that use the Biosense DMR system to test the safety, feasibility, and efficacy of the left ventricular mapped DMR approach.[17] Groups of patients include those with chronic refractory ischemia who are poor candidates for either angioplasty or coronary bypass surgical procedures. Phase I safety and feasibility studies have recently been completed in the USA and Europe. In the USA, Biosense guided percutaneous laser revascularization has been successful in 77 patients. Procedural success was achieved in 76 (99%) of 77 patients. One patient had pericardial effusion and underwent pericardiocentesis, and one patient developed minor stroke. Immediate results did not show any change on surface electrocardiography. Minor CK-MB elevations (<3 times normal) occurred in 22% of the patients, and moderate rise (3–8 times normal) occurred in only 4% of the patients. The left ventricular ejection fraction did not change immediately or at 1 month after the procedure. Improvement in exercise times (387 to 453 s) was significant (p < 0.001), and improvement in CCS class occurred in most patients (3.3 to 2.0 at 3 and 6 months, p < 0.001). Similar results were reported in 35 patients using the Biosense system in phase I registries at three sites in Europe. Representative electromechanical guided DMR cases in the anterior wall and the inferior wall are shown in Figures 6.7 and 6.8, respectively. The laser catheter-tip location and orientation are presented on the

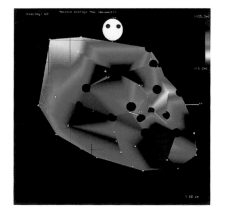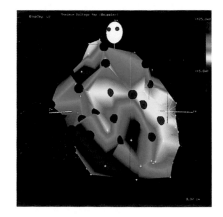

**Figure 6.7:** *Representative case of percutaneous DMR using the Biosense system. Electroanatomical maps (right oblique and left oblique projections in the left and right panels, respectively) follow a catheter-based DMR done in the anterior and septal zones. The laser sites were tagged on the map (brown dots) in real time to show the exact endocardial location and precise distances of 29 laser channels in the treated areas.*

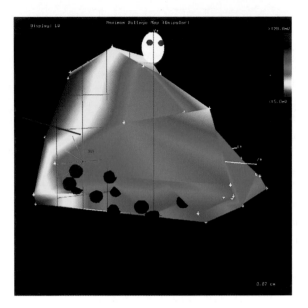

*Figure 6.8:* Representative case of percutaneous DMR using the Biosense left ventricular endocardial mapping system in a patient with severe angina and previous coronary artery bypass surgery. Electroanatomical maps (right oblique projection) follow a catheter-based DMR done in the inferior zone. The laser sites were tagged on the map (brown dots) in real time to show the exact endocardial location and precise distances of 14 laser channels in the treated areas. The map colors show the extent of endocardial voltage potentials, signifying preserved myocardial viability in the treated zones.

map, and the exact channel location is tagged on the left ventricle map in real time, immediately after laser activation.

A randomized "blinded" phase II clinical study (DIRECT = DMR In Regeneration of Endomyocardial Channels Trial) is underway in the USA to test the clinical efficacy of percutaneous Biosense guided DMR versus left ventricle electromechanical mapping without laser activation. A randomized phase II clinical study (Euro-DIRECT) is underway in Europe comparing Biosense guided DMR against "best" attempted medical therapy.

## Future directions

New approaches for catheter-based intramyocardial therapy ("pharmacological" DMR) are undergoing development to achieve endomyocardial injection of therapeutic agents such as angiogenic growth factors, genes, or both. The use of

Biosense electromechanical guided mapping technology would allow precise localization of the catheter within the left ventricle, and accurately identify target sites for injection of local pharmacotherapy. Using the Biosense guidance system, we have shown that transgenes can be transfected into designated myocardial sites.[13] This less-invasive catheter-based system may offer a clear advantage over surgically based transepicardial injection approaches for intramyocardial angiogenic therapy.

## Acknowledgement

The pathological work and scientific contributions of Dr Christian C Haudenschild are gratefully acknowledged.

## References

1.  Ben-Haim SA, Osadchy D, Schuster I et al. Nonfluoroscopic, *in vivo* navigation and mapping technology. *Nature Med* 1996; **2:** 1393–5.

2.  Gepstein L, Ben-Haim SA. 3D cardiac imaging of electromechanical coupling. *Adv Exp Med Biol* 1997; **430:** 303–11.

3.  Gepstein L, Hayam G, Ben-Haim SA. A novel method for nonfluoroscopic catheter-based electroanatomical mapping of the heart. In vitro and in vivo accuracy results. *Circulation* 1997; **95:** 1611–22.

4.  Gepstein L, Hayam G, Shpun S, Ben-Haim SA. Hemodynamic evaluation of the heart with a nonfluoroscopic electromechanical mapping technique. *Circulation* 1997; **96:** 3672–80.

5.  Shpun S, Gepstein L, Hayam G, Ben-Haim SA. Guidance of radiofrequency endocardial ablation with real-time three-dimensional magnetic navigation system. *Circulation* 1997; **96:** 2016–21.

6.  Kornowski R, Hong MK, Gepstein L et al. Preliminary animal and clinical experiences using an electro-mechanical endocardial mapping procedure to distinguish infarcted from healthy myocardium. *Circulation* 1998; **98:** 1116–24.

7.  Gepstein L, Goldin A, Lessick L et al. Electromechanical characterization of chronic myocardial infarction in the canine coronary occlusion mode. *Circulation* 1998; **98:** 2055–64.

8.  Kornowski R, Hong MK, Leon MB. Comparison between left ventricular electro-mechanical mapping and radionuclide perfusion imaging for detection of myocardial viability. *Circulation* 1998; **98:** 1837–41.

9.  Shah DC, Jais P, Haissaguerre M et al. Three-dimensional mapping of the common atrial flutter circuit in the right atrium. *Circulation* 1997; **96:** 3904–12.

10. Kottkamp H, Hindricks G, Breithardt G, Borggrefe M. Three-dimensional electromagnetic catheter technology: electroanatomical mapping of the right atrium and ablation of ectopic atrial tachycardia. *J Cardiovasc Electrophysiol* 1997; **8:** 1332–7.

11. Smeets JLRM, Ben-Haim SA, Rodriguez LM et al. New method for nonfluoroscopic endocardial mapping in humans. *Circulation* 1998; **97:** 2426–32.

12. Kornowski R, Hong MK, Haudenschild C et al. Feasibility and safety of percutaneous direct myocardial revascularization using Biosense™ system in porcine hearts. *Coronary Artery Dis* 1998; **9:** 535–40.

13. Kornowski R, Fuchs S, Vodocotz Y et al. Successful gene transfer in a porcine ischemia model using the Biosense guided transendocardial injection catheter. *J Am Coll Cardiol* 1999; **33:** 354A.

14. Kornowski R, Hong MK, Leon MB. Current perspectives on direct myocardial revascularization. *Am J Cardiol* 1998; **81:** 44–8E.

15. Kornowski R, Hong MH, Haudenschild CC, Leon MB. Potentially hazardous effects of high-power holmium:YAG lasers during direct myocardial revascularization in porcine hearts. *Am J Cardiol* 1997; **80** (suppl 7A): 14S.

16. Haudenschild CC, Bastaki M, Boenigk K et al. Angiogenesis in response to minimal laser injury in porcine myocardium. *J Am Coll Cardiol* 1998; **31:** 307A.

17. Kornowski R, Moses J, Baim D et al. Percutaneous direct myocardial revascularization guided by Biosense left ventricular mapping in patients with refractory coronary ischemia. *J Am Coll Cardiol* 1999; **33:** 354A.

# 7. Percutaneous Transluminal Myocardial Revascularization (PTMR): The Eclipse System and Studies

Gregg W Stone

Nearly 1 million patients in the USA alone undergo percutaneous intervention or coronary artery bypass grafting every year for manifest atherosclerotic coronary artery disease, often with dramatic improvements in symptoms. Nonetheless, many patients who present with ischemic heart disease are inadequately addressed by these measures, including those with myocardial territories that are non-revascularizable with current techniques, or in whom angioplasty results in incessant restenosis, or for whom surgery carries excessive risk. For these patients, transmyocardial revascularization (TMR) promises to provide symptom relief to the vast majority. Studies have shown that about 70% of patients with class III–IV angina have marked reduction in chest pain with the surgical creation of myocardial channels with a $CO_2$ or holmium:YAG laser.[1-4] Unfortunately, however, the surgical approach in these high-risk patients has been associated with a 10–20% early mortality,[1-3] prompting the development of less invasive, potentially safer, percutaneous methods.

Three manufacturers have developed percutaneous catheter-based systems for transmyocardial revascularization, all of which use holmium:YAG laser energy carried by fiberoptic cables to create myocardial channels photoacoustically. This chapter will describe the percutaneous transluminal myocardial revascularization (PTMR) system developed by Eclipse Surgical Technologies, Inc (Sunnyvale, CA), and will discuss completed and ongoing clinical trials of this device.

## The Eclipse PTMR system and technique

The Eclipse energy source is a solid-state, mid-infrared (wavelength 2.1 microns) pulsed holmium:YAG (yttrium-aluminium-garnet) laser with average 20 W peak power (Figure 7.1). The current device has a fixed pulsewidth of 200 ms and a pulse rate of 5 hz. The unit has a small footprint and minimal warm-up time. Each multifiber laser catheter (SlimFlex) is recognized by the console, and is individually tuned and calibrated to deliver predictable and uniform energy output.

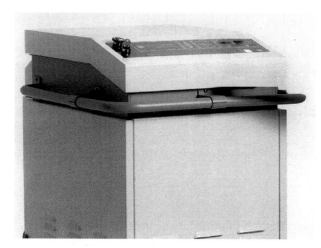

**Figure 7.1:** *The Eclipse solid-state holmium:YAG laser console.*

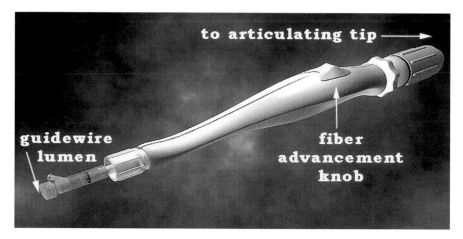

**Figure 7.2:** *The multifunction control handle attaches to the proximal end of the guide catheter, allowing axial translational and rotational control of the catheter and laser fiber.*

The Eclipse PTMR procedure is performed as follows: after the insertion of a 9F arterial sheath, 5000–7500 units intravenous heparin is given to maintain the ACT at about 250 s. Standard conscious sedation is used. The left ventricle is entered retrograde across the aortic valve with a standard pigtail catheter. Biplane left ventriculography is then done for road-mapping. The pigtail catheter is withdrawn over an exchange length guidewire and replaced with a steerable

**78**

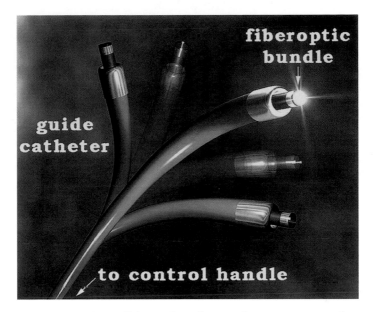

*Figure 7.3:* *The distal tip of the guide catheter is shown, containing the multifiber laser bundle. The distal tip of the guide can articulate about 90 degrees in any direction. Activating the fiber advancement knob on the control panel advances the laser fiber approximately 3 mm into the myocardium.*

PTMR guide catheter, which is manufactured in 5 cm (shorter) and 7 cm (longer) versions. After removal of the guidewire, the proximal end of the guide catheter is joined to a multifunction control handle, containing a central lumen for the guidewire or laser bundle, articulation ring, and laser fiber advancement knob (Figure 7.2). The multifiber laser bundle is then passed into the central lumen, and aligned with the distal tip of the guide catheter. By axially advancing and retracting the guide catheter, and articulating its distal tip with the control ring, the guide catheter can be directed against any myocardial surface using biplane fluoroscopic control (Figure 7.3).

Contact with the myocardium is confirmed by visual feedback and tactile sensation. Once proper position is established and the catheter is stable (no ectopy), the laser is activated by a foot pedal while the operator simultaneously advances the fiber bundle. Five pulses are delivered during each run; the first two are "dummy pulses", and the next three are active. The fiber is advanced 3 mm into the myocardium during which tissue is photoacoustically ablated; a mechanical stop arrests further advancement (Figure 7.4). Myocardial ablation is typically recognized by the occurrence of 1–2 PVCs during fiber advancement

**79**

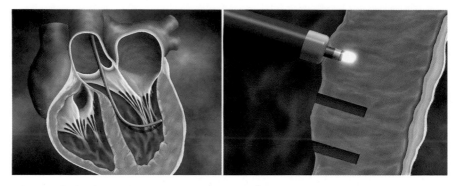

*Figure 7.4: The guide catheter sites retrograde across the aortic valve against the myocardium (left panel). Advancement of the laser bundle 3 mm into the myocardium, together with laser activation, creates tissue channels about 5 mm in depth, or slightly greater than half the thickness of the left ventricular myocardium (right panel).*

and laser activation. In-vitro data have shown that this technique results in a channel depth of about 5 mm $\pm$ 1 mm.

After the creation of a single channel, the laser fiber is retracted and the guide repositioned to a different location in the same myocardial territory, about 1 cm away, and the process is repeated. About 10–15 channels are created per major myocardial territory (anterior, inferior, or lateral walls). The septum may also be ablated. The apex of the left ventricle, however, is typically avoided because natural thinning increases the risk of perforation.

After the learning curve is scaled, the entire procedure typically takes 30–45 min, including 15 min of fluoroscopy. The PTMR procedure is usually painless; occasionally patients will describe a "warm sensation" as the laser is activated. Pleuritic chest or shoulder pain suggests perforation, and needs immediate echocardiography. As described below, perforations occur infrequently, and are usually though not always inconsequential. In the absence of complications, patients may be discharged later the same day or on the following morning after the PTMR procedure.

## Advantages and disadvantages of PTMR

Compared with surgical TMR, the PTMR procedure offers several advantages. It is clearly less invasive and therefore inherently safer, minimal anticoagulation is required, general anesthesia is not needed, and surgical incisions and cardiopulmonary bypass are avoided. PTMR offers the capability to treat the septum and posterior wall, which are regions generally not approachable by the surgical technique. The patient recovers more quickly after PTMR than TMR, and in most cases is able to be discharged the next day, resulting in a shorter, less expensive hospital stay with earlier return to work. The relative ease and safety of PTMR allows multiple treatment sessions, if necessary.

Several drawbacks of the percutaneous approach should be acknowledged, however. PTMR requires retrograde cannulation of the aortic valve, and therefore cannot be done in patients with moderate or severe aortic stenosis or an aortic valve prosthesis. Aortic valve injury is also theoretically possible. Unlike with TMR, the heart is in motion, which can make it difficult to obtain stable catheter position. Ventricular arrhythmias are common, especially in small cavity left ventricles such as in patients with hypertension. Hypertrophied papillary muscles can make lasing of the inferoposterolateral walls difficult. Guide catheter manipulation can dislodge aortic debris or mural thrombi, resulting in cerebrovascular or other thromboembolic events.

Possibly most importantly, precise positioning of the laser fiber bundle is difficult since the percutaneous approach uses fluoroscopic guidance alone (though the clinical relevance and necessity of exact positioning remains uncertain). This may result in lack of channel uniformity and wall coverage, doubt as to whether or not channels were even formed, and the risk of creating multiple channels in the same location (the "channel on channel" phenomenon), hypothetically increasing the risk of perforation.

Finally, TMR, by definition, creates transmural channels, which is, of course, of no clinical consequence since the surgical technique involves pericardial incision. By contrast, the inadvertent creation of truly transmyocardial channels with the percutaneous approach, if not self-sealing, may result in hemodynamic compromise or frank tamponade requiring emergency pericardiocentesis or surgical repair.

## Candidates for PTMR

It has been estimated that more than 200 000 patients per year might benefit from PTMR in the USA alone. Most of the investigation of PTMR has thus far been focused on the "no option" patient – the patient with medically refractory class III–IV angina and no or little chance for relief with standard percutaneous or surgical revascularization methods. This category includes: patients with diffuse atherosclerotic disease or with small target vessels; those with chronic total occlusions with either unseen, small or diseased distal targets; those with incessant restenosis after angioplasty with undesirable surgical alternatives; patients who have had one or more previous bypass operations and have severe saphenous vein graft degeneration, with or without a patent left internal mammary artery conduit; and patients with diffuse transplant vasculopathy.

Despite encouraging initial studies with PTMR in no-option patients, as described below, it may turn out that PTMR will most frequently be applied in the future as part of a "hybrid" procedure, in which percutaneous intervention is done together with laser myocardial revascularization. Two scenarios can be envisioned for this approach. In the first (and likely to become the most common), angioplasty is done in one or more myocardial territories, followed by PTMR in different and remote non-revascularizable zones. In the second, percutaneous intervention and PTMR may be done in the same myocardial territory. This may be advantageous for the patient in whom restenosis is likely (eg, >50% risk) after angioplasty or stenting, the theory being that PTMR-induced angiogenesis may ameliorate the signs or symptoms of recurrent ischemia otherwise expected with restenosis of an epicardial coronary artery.

## Clinical (human) studies of PTMR with the Eclipse system

### Pilot studies

Overall, the Eclipse PTMR system has been used in more than 800 patients worldwide. Much of the early work with Eclipse PTMR was done by Fayaz Shawl and Bill Knopf outside the USA.[6,7] Detailed reports of the safety and efficacy of this device are just recently being presented. Before phase II randomized trials, the safety of Eclipse PTMR was examined by collating reports from 176 consecutive patients, including 111 "no-option" patients undergoing PTMR alone, and 65 patients undergoing hybrid procedures. The 111 no-option patients consisted of 25 cases from US phase I registries, 39 cases from phase II training or lead-in patients, and 47 cases from outside the US monitored by the company. The 65 hybrid patients were comprised of 27 patients from a phase I registry that assessed the outcomes of PTMR in patients at high risk for restenosis, plus 38 patients in which angioplasty and PTMR were done in different myocardial territories, either in phase I studies or lead-in cases in phase II.

The overall safety data from these 176 patients are shown in Table 7.1. Major adverse periprocedural events occurred in six (3.4%) patients, including five deaths. One no-option patient had an uncomplicated PTMR, but without relief from symptoms. He died after a palliative bypass surgery. A second no-option patient also had an uncomplicated but unsuccessful PTMR procedure; PTMR was repeated on a compassionate use basis, and the patient died from multisystem failure. The other three deaths were in patients undergoing hybrid PTMR. In the first, the guide catheter caused a left main dissection, and the patient expired

**Table 7.1  Periprocedural adverse events after PTMR in 176 patients**

| | |
|---|---|
| Major adverse events | |
| Death | 5 (2.9%) |
| Emergency CABG | 1 (0.6%) |
| MI (CPK > 3× nl) | 3 (1.7%) |
| Any MACE | 6 (3.4%) |
| Other adverse events | |
| Pericardial effusion | 11 (6.3%) |
| Pericardiocentesis | 3 (1.7%) |
| Tamponade | 1 (0.6%) |
| Ventricular tachycardia (cardioverted) | 1 (0.6%) |
| Complete heart block (resolved) | 1 (0.6%) |
| Hypotension (requiring IABP) | 1 (0.6%) |
| Atrial fibrillation (post procedure, cardioverted) ) | 1 (0.6%) |
| Transient ischemic attack (post procedure, resolved) ) | 1 (0.6%) |

CABG = coronary artery bypass grafting
MI = myocardial infarction
MACE = major adverse cardiac events (death, CABG, MI)
IABP = intra-aortic balloon counterpulsation

without the laser being fired. In the second, the procedure was uncomplicated, but the patient developed a massive myocardial infarction from subacute stent closure, and died. The final patient was a true laser related death: the PTMR guide catheter perforated the left ventricular myocardium, resulting in tamponade that needed surgical repair. The patient survived this but developed stent closure immediately postoperatively, resulting in a massive MI and ventricular free wall rupture from this event, not in the laser territory per se.

Thus, given the early experience that these cases represent, together with the high-risk nature of the patients and the fact that most of the deaths were not directly related to the PTMR procedure, the relatively high rate of major adverse cardiac events may be understandable. The 6.3% rate of pericardial effusions, however, is notable. Most of these presented as minor or moderate pleuritic chest or shoulder pain, with a small effusion discerned by echocardiography. The patients remained hemodynamically stable, and their pain typically resolved within several hours to a day at most. Of the 11 effusions noted, however, three were large and needed pericardiocentesis, and one resulted in tamponade and need for surgical repair.

The causes of pericardial effusions (ie, myocardial perforations) after PTMR are multifactorial. Perforation is typically caused by the laser catheter, most frequently due to excessive mechanical pressure applied to the guide catheter resulting in thinned myocardium before the laser is fired. If extreme, frank guide catheter perforation of the left ventricular free wall can occur, as demonstrated at surgery in one case. The presently available guide catheter is relatively inflexible and potentially traumatic, and some of the tactile feel required for optimal safety is lost in the adhesion between the introducer sheath and guide catheter. Thus, reduction in the presently observed rate of perforation will probably await future improvements in equipment, and improved operator technique and experience. In this regard, it is critical for the interventionalist to avoid akinetic and scarred myocardial zones. For this reason, transthoracic echocardiography is now routinely done before PTMR, with lasing allowed only in regions with an echocardiographic thickness of ≥9 mm. Future technical innovations, including EKG gating, on-line IVUS guidance,[5] and tailored energy and pulse parameter selection will also increase the safety of PTMR.

*1) No-option patients*
Whitlow and co-workers have recently reported the detailed results of PTMR in 41 no-option patients with class III–IV angina at seven centers.[8,9] Mean age was 62 ± 8 years, 85% were men, mean LVEF was 42% ± 11, and mean angina class was 3.7 ± 0.5. The baseline high-risk nature of the population was reflected in the fact that 68% of patients had undergone prior CABG, 61% prior PTCA, 76% had triple vessel disease, and 63% had prior myocardial infarction. The mean total procedure time was 61 ± 23 min (including laser time of 20 ± 13 min); 17 ± 5 myocardial laser channels were created per patient. No periprocedural major adverse events occurred. Patients were discharged 2.0 ± 1.5 days post procedure. Over the next 6 months one patient developed a non Q-wave MI, one patient developed a Q-wave MI, and two patients died (one after repeat compassionate-use PTMR, one after compassionate palliative CABG). One patient underwent PTCA; no other revascularization procedures were done. Dramatic relief of angina was reported in most patients; angina relief by ≥2 classes was present in 80% of patients at 3 months, and 85% of patients at 6 months (Figure 7.5). Baseline Naughton exercise treadmill time was 250 ± 144 s before PTMR, and 500 ± 208 s at 6 months (p < 0.05). In a separate report, Shawl and colleagues[10] described similar results in 27 patients from two hospitals in India and Maryland.

**84**

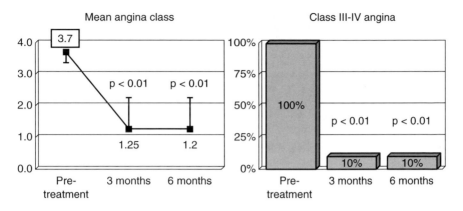

**Figure 7.5:** *Angina class in 41 no-option patients before PTMR, and at 3 and 6 months after PTMR. The mean angina class is displayed in the left panel, and the proportion of patients with class III–IV angina is shown in the right panel.*

From these studies,[8–10] the following conclusions may be drawn: PTMR may be done safely in high-risk "no-option" patients with an acceptable complication rate; the degree of angina relief (and accompanying improved exercise tolerance) is often dramatic, typically occurs within the first 3 months, and is sustained to 6 months; given the lack of a defined mechanism of PTMR, the absence of demonstrable relief of ischemia in many patients, and the possible role of denervation or the placebo effect, phase II randomized trials are required to establish the usefulness of PTMR alone in patients with class III–IV angina and no percutaneous or surgical alternatives.

*2) Hybrid patients at high risk for restenosis.*
Stone and coworkers reported the results of a pilot phase I study at five sites of 27 patients with class III–IV angina undergoing percutaneous intervention of one or more lesion(s) at high risk for restenosis plus PTMR in the same myocardial territories to ameliorate recurrent ischemia should restenosis occur.[11] Entry criteria included patients with diabetes, and lesions in vessels with reference diameter of less than 3.0 mm, lesion length of more than 15 mm, ostial lesions, chronic total occlusions, bifurcation lesions, saphenous vein grafts, and multiple lesion angioplasty. Mean age was 63 ± 10 years; 74% were men, 33% had diabetes, 67% had triple vessel disease, 28% had prior heart failure, 44% had prior MI, and all but one patient had undergone prior revascularization (including prior PTCA in 89% of patients and prior bypass surgery in 67%). Intravenous nitroglycerin was being administered to 37% of patients at the time of the procedure.

**Table 7.2 Major adverse cardiac events 6 months after percutaneous intervention plus PTMR in 27 patients**

| Major adverse events | |
| --- | --- |
| Death | 5 (18.5%) |
| early | 3 (11.1%) |
| late | 2 (7.4%) |
| Q-wave myocardial infarction | 2 (7.4%) |
| Target vessel revascularization | 5 (18.5%) |
| PTCA | 3 (11.1%) |
| CABG | 2 (7.4%) |
| Angina class | |
| Class III–IV angina | |
| pretreatment | 100% |
| 3 months | 19% |
| 6 months | 12% |

Stents were implanted in 42% of patients, rotational or laser atherectomy was done in 19%, and balloon angioplasty was done in 96% of patients. Successful percutaneous intervention was achieved in 26 (96%) patients, after which PTMR was attempted. A mean number of $17 \pm 6$ channels were created per patient. Total procedure time was $96 \pm 77$ min; the duration of PTMR was $19 \pm 12$ min. Major adverse cardiac events within the first month of the procedure occurred in three (11.1%) patients, including, as described above, one patient who died after a left main dissection in whom the laser was never fired. In the remaining 26 patients who actually underwent PTMR, major adverse events within 30 days occurred in two patients (7.7%), including one death from subacute stent closure related to a distal dissection 24 h after the procedure (no laser complication noted), and one death from guide catheter rupture of the myocardium, as previously described. Myocardial infarction, defined as CPK-MB of more than $3\times$ normal occurred in 18.8% of patients, including two patients (7.4%) with Q-wave infarction. Only one (4.8%) of 22 patients with CPK data

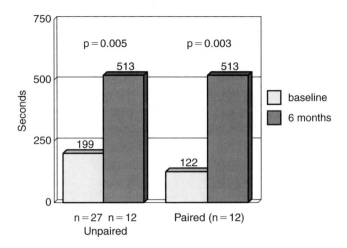

*Figure 7.6:* Naughton exercise test data in 27 patients undergoing percutaneous intervention + PTMR in 27 patients with lesions at high risk for restenosis. (Note: exercise time was imputed to 0 s if the patient was unable to exercise.)

developed a total CPK of more than 150 IU/ml. Pericardial effusions were noted in three (11.1%) patients, including the single patient with tamponade. No patient had a hemorrhagic or neurological complication. The mean hospital stay post procedure was 1.8 ± 1.5 days.

Cumulative clinical results at 6 months (including the in-hospital phase) are shown in Table 7.2, and pre-trial and 6 month exercise data appear in Figure 7.6. Two late deaths occurred: one patient died in his sleep of unclear causes 124 days after discharge, and one patient died of stent occlusion at 90 days.

From that study[11], the following conclusions can be drawn: acutely formed PTMR channels may not be protective from severe ischemia if the epicardial vessel acutely closes (consistent with the canine data from Whitaker et al[12]); the high mortality in this small series most probably reflects the learning curve, technical issues to be overcome, and patient selection; symptomatic restenosis can still occur despite PTMR having been done in the same myocardial territory; whether or not PTMR can ameliorate symptoms in patients with only moderate restenosis remains speculative, and would require a randomized trial with angiographic follow-up for determination.

## Phase II randomized trials

On the basis of the above pilot studies, three phase II randomized trials were begun with the Eclipse PTMR system. Inclusion criteria were similar in all three studies: class III–IV angina refractory to medication, LVEF 30%, demonstrable viable myocardium in the treatment zone(s), with echocardiographic demonstration of wall thickness ⩾9 mm in the treatment areas. Similarly, the exclusion criteria were also shared: congestive heart failure class ⩾2, aortic stenosis with a valve area of less than 1 cm$^2$ (or aortic valve prosthesis), inability to exercise pre-procedure unless due to severe class IV angina, electrocardiographic left bundle branch block, WPW syndrome or left ventricular hypertrophy precluding the diagnosis of ischemia, left ventricular aneurysm, evidence of mural thrombus or recent myocardial infarction within 3 months, dilated or tortuous aorta, and other severe co-morbid conditions making it unlikely that the patient would complete follow-up.


*PTMR versus maximal medical therapy in no-option patients*
In this study, 335 patients with refractory class III–IV angina on maximal medical therapy with no percutaneous or surgical options for revascularization were prospectively randomized at 20 US centers to PTMR versus continued conservative care. All patients had to have demonstrable ischemia with a positive functional test if able to exercise. The primary endpoint was improvement in exercise test duration from baseline to 12 months. The *preliminary results* of this study were reported for the first time by Pat Whitlow from the Cleveland Clinic at the 48th Annual Scientific Sessions of the American College of Cardiology in New Orleans, LA, on March 8th, 1999.

PTMR was done in 169 patients. A mean of 19 ± 7 channels were created per patient during a procedure lasting 86 ± 46 min. Laser time was 23 ± 13 min. Procedural success without complications was reported in 95.8% of patients. Major procedural complications included one death (0.6%), five cases (3%) of tamponade, one stroke (0.6%), six non Q-wave myocardial infarctions (3.6%), but no Q-wave infarctions.

The angina-class improvement at 3 months in each group is shown in Table 7.3. Overall, angina improvement of ⩾2 classes from baseline to 3 months was noted in 50% of patients undergoing PTMR versus 17% of control patients (p < 0.0001). Among PTMR patients, exercise time increased from an average of 381 s at baseline to 529 s at 3 months (p < 0.0002). By contrast, there was no improvement in exercise tolerance from baseline to 3 months in patients not undergoing PTMR (mean 424 *vs* 415 s, respectively, p = NS). Cumulative clinical events to 3 months are shown in Figure 7.7, and were similar between the two groups. Readmission to hospital after discharge within the first 3 months was needed in 33.6% of patients undergoing PTMR versus 36.0% of controls (p = NS). Thus, these early data suggest that PTMR with the Eclipse system may be done safely in patients with severe angina and no alternative pathways for revascularization, resulting in marked symptom benefit in an additional one-third

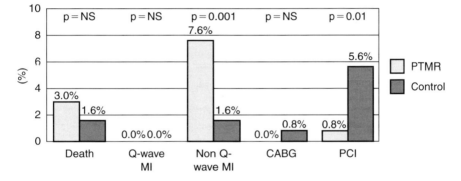

**Table 7.3 Angina class at 3 months in 335 "no-option" patients randomly assigned PTMR versus conservative care**

Canadian Cardiovascular Classification

|  | PTMR | Control |
|---|---|---|
| Number | 169 | 166 |
| No improvement | 19% | 47% |
| Improvement by 1 angina grade | 31% | 36% |
| Improvement by ≥2 angina grades | 50% | 17% |

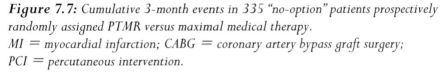

*Figure 7.7:* Cumulative 3-month events in 335 "no-option" patients prospectively randomly assigned PTMR versus maximal medical therapy.
MI = myocardial infarction; CABG = coronary artery bypass graft surgery; PCI = percutaneous intervention.

of patients compared with maximal medical therapy. Overall improved exercise tolerance may be shown as early as 3 months after the procedure. The 6- and 12-month results from this important trial are presently being collected to assess whether these early results are durable.

*Hybrid PTMR in patients undergoing percutaneous intervention*
Two prospective multicenter randomized trials are underway enrolling patients in whom angioplasty and PTMR are done during the same procedure. In the first study at 40 sites, 750 patients undergoing successful percutaneous intervention of one or more epicardial coronary arteries, who also have additional non-revascularizable myocardial zones are being randomly assigned to either

percutaneous intervention plus PTMR of these territories or angioplasty alone. An example of a suitable patient might be the patient with a totally occluded right coronary artery in whom stenting is successful in the left anterior distribution. Patients are given heavy sedation in an attempt to blind them to whether or not PTMR was done after angioplasty. A questionnaire at the time of discharge will assess each patient's belief of treatment assignment. The primary endpoint of this study is improvement in exercise duration at 12 months. Rates of restenosis will be controlled for in an angiographic substudy in 250 patients at 6 months.

The second trial at 20 sites includes 140 patients with chronic total occlusions who have undergone an unsuccessful but uncomplicated angioplasty attempt at recanalization, and in whom the standard of care would be medical therapy (eg, patients with single vessel disease). Patients are being randomly assigned to PTMR of the myocardium subtended by the totally occluded vessel or conservative medical management. Again, the primary endpoint of this study is improvement in exercise duration at 12 months compared with baseline.

## The Eclipse PTMR system — conclusions and perspectives for future use

Available data suggest that the Eclipse PTMR system may have a valuable role in the care of patients with severe coronary artery disease with few or no viable alternatives for revascularization. Given the dire condition of many of these patients, and the inordinate amount of scarce resources they consume, any method that gives even relief from symptoms is welcome. It is notable that the reduction in angina scores afforded by Eclipse PTMR, as shown in the no-option randomized trial, was mirrored in the results of the randomized PACIFIC trial (Potential Anginal Class Improvement From Intramyocardial Channels), which used the CardioGenesis percutaneous myocardial revascularization (PMR) system,[13] a holmium:YAG pulsed laser that also relies on fluoroscopic guidance. Furthermore, it is clear that PTMR can be done more safely than its surgical TMR counterpart, while apparently affording similar degrees of relief from symptoms. The role of PTMR as part of a hybrid procedure in patients undergoing percutaneous intervention is less well established, and is the subject of ongoing investigation.

For PTMR to become widely accepted, several hurdles remain to be overcome. Importantly, the mechanism through which laser myocardial revascularization produces anginal relief must be clarified. It is now accepted by most investigators that the freshly created myocardial channels fibrose and close entirely within several weeks of the procedure.[14,15] Thus, chronically patent sinusoids supplying endocardial blood flow, as originally hypothesized after examination of the reptilian heart model,[16,17] cannot explain long-term symptomatic benefit. While photoacoustic laser induction of the creation of new blood vessels over the first 1–2 months after the procedure (angiogenesis) is felt by many to be the most likely explanation for patient improvement from PTMR,[18–21] other theories, including myocardial blood flow redistribution, denervation,[22,23] and the placebo effect, have been postulated. Indeed, it has been difficult to show reduction in ischemia after TMR or PTMR with routine non-invasive testing with isotopes such as thallium, though newer techniques, such as dobutamine stress echocardiography, myocardial contrast echocardiography, and positron emission tomography have shown improved perfusion in selected patients.[24,25] It is possible that PTMR provides subtle improvements in endocardial blood flow that require more sensitive tools for detection.

Finally, as previously discussed, major improvements in equipment are required to make the PTMR procedure safer and more effective. In this regard, it is notable that Eclipse and CardioGenesis have recently completed a worldwide merger. It is anticipated that the combination of intellectual property and engineering resources will allow rapid technological advancements to be produced from this merger, resulting in more flexible and steerable guide catheters, real-time IVUS guidance, and selectable variable pulse and energy parameters, to name but a few. If the results of the recently completed, ongoing, and planned randomized trials continue to be positive, it is anticipated that the Eclipse PTMR system may soon become an accepted and possibly indispensable device in the interventionalist's toolbox.

## References

1. Horvath KA, Cohn LH, Cooley DA et al. Transmyocardial laser revascularization: results of a multicenter trial with transmyocardial laser revascularization used as sole therapy for end-stage coronary artery disease. *J Thorac Cardiovasc Surg* 1997; **113:** 645–54.

2. Cooley DA, Frazier OH, Kadipasaoglu KA et al. Transmyocardial laser revascularization: clinical experience with twelve month follow-up. *J Thorac Cardiovasc Surg* 1996; **111:** 791–9.

3. Allen KB, Fudge TL, Schoettle GP et al. Prospective randomized multicenter trial of transmyocardial revascularization versus maximal medical management in patients with refractory class IV angina: 12 month results. *Circulation* 1998; **98:** I-476.

4. Dowling RD, Allen KB, Fudge T et al. Recent experience of transmyocardial revascularization in a prospective randomized trial demonstrates dramatic symptom relief and excellent safety profile. *J Am Coll Cardiol* 1999; **33:** 380A.

5.  O'Neill WW, Grube E, de Swart H, Bar F. Feasibility study of percutaneous transmyocardial revascularization with forward-looking A-mode ultrasound for real-time wall-thickness measurements. *J Am Coll Cardiol* 1999; **33:** 101A.

6.  Shawl FA, Kaul U, Singh B, Rigali G. Percutaneous transluminal myocardial revascularization (PTMR): procedural results and early clinical outcome. *J Am Coll Cardiol* 1998; **31:** 223A.

7.  Knopf W, Londero H, Kaul U et al. Feasibility study of percutaneous transluminal myocardial revascularization (PTMR) with a holmium laser and fiberoptic delivery system. *J Am Coll Cardiol* 1998; **31:** 235A.

8.  Whitlow PL, Knopf WD, O'Neill WW et al. Percutaneous transmyocardial revascularization in patients with refractory angina. *Circulation* 1998; **98:** I-87.

9.  Whitlow PL, Knopf WD, O'Neill WW et al. Six month follow-up of percutaneous transmyocardial revascularization in patients with refractory angina. *J Am Coll Cardiol* 1999; **33:** 29A.

10. Shawl FA, Domanski MJ, Kaul U et al. Procedural results and early clinical outcome of percutaneous transluminal myocardial revascularization. *Am J Cardiol* 1999; **83:** 498–501.

11. Stone GW, Shawl FA, Taussig A et al. Percutaneous myocardial laser revascularization in patients with class III–IV angina and lesions at high risk for restenosis – results of the phase I pilot study as a preamble to a large, randomized trial. *Circulation* 1998; **98:** I-557.

12. Whitaker P, Kloner RA, Przyklenk K. Laser-mediated myocardial channels do not salvage acutely ischemic myocardium. *J Am Coll Cardiol* 1993; **22:** 302–9.

13. Oesterle SN, Yeung A, Ali N et al. The CardioGenesis percutaneous myocardial revascularization (PMR) randomized trial: initial clinical results. *J Am Coll Cardiol* 1999; **33:** 380A.

14. Hardy RI, James FW, Millard RW, Kaplan S. Regional myocardial blood flow and cardiac mechanics in dog hearts with $CO_2$ laser induced intramyocardial revascularization. *Basic Res Cardiol* 1990; **85:** 179–97.

15. Kohmoto T, Fischer PE, Gu A et al. Does blood flow through holmium:YAG transmyocardial laser channels? *Ann Thorac Surg* 1996; **61:** 861–8.

16. Khomoto T, Argenziano M, Yamamoto N et al. Assessment of transmyocardial perfusion in alligator hearts. *Circulation* 1997; **95:** 1585–91.

17. Whittaker P, Kloner RA. Transmural channels as a source of blood flow to ischemic myocardium: insights from the reptilian heart. *Circulation* 1997; **95:** 1357–9.

18. Mack CA, Magovern CJ, Hahn RT et al. Channel patency and neovascularization after transmyocardial revascularization using an excimer laser: results and comparisons to nonlased channels. *Circulation* 1997; **96:** II-65–9.

19. Chu V, Giaid A, Kuang J et al. Transmyocardial laser revascularization induced angiogenic response. *J Am Coll Cardiol* 1999; **33:** 342A.

20. Kohmoto T, DeRosa CM, Yamamoto N et al. Evidence of vascular growth associated with laser treatment of normal canine myocardium. *Ann Thorac Surg* 1998; **65:** 1360–7.

21. Yamamoto N, Kohmoto T, Gu A et al. Angiogenesis is enhanced in ischemic canine myocardium by transmural laser revascularization. *J Am Coll Cardiol* 1998; **31:** 1426–33.

22. Stoll HP, Hutchins GD, Fain RL et al. Transmyocardial laser revascularization (TMR) induces regional myocardial denervation. *Circulation* 1998; **98:** I-349.

23. Kwong KF, Kanellopoulos GK, Nickols JC et al. Transmyocardial laser treatment denervates canine myocardium. *J Thorac Cardiovasc Surg* 1997; **114:** 883–9.

24. Stahl F, Lauer B, Junghans U et al. Increased myocardial glucose-uptake after percutaneous myocardial laser revascularization in patients with end-stage coronary artery disease. *J Am Coll Cardiol* 1999; **33:** 335A.

25. Donovan CL, Landolfo KP, Hughes GC et al. Improvement in inducible ischemia during dobutamine stress echocardiography after transmyocardial laser revascularization in patients with refractory angina pectoris. *J Am Coll Cardiol* 1997; **30:** 607–12.

# 8. THE CARDIOGENESIS™ PERCUTANEOUS MYOCARDIAL REVASCULARIZATION SYSTEM

Robert J Whitbourn and Stephen N Oesterle

## Introduction

In patients with coronary artery disease, improvements in myocardial perfusion have traditionally been achieved by methods that increase blood flow through the existing coronary vessels. By contrast, percutaneous myocardial revascularization (PMR) uses laser energy transmitted to the endocardial surface of the left ventricle along a flexible, fiberoptic catheter, via a femoral artery.

Delivered energy vaporizes myocardial tissue, creating channels from the endocardial surface into the targeted area of ischemic myocardium. The thermal, mechanical, and chemical effects of this laser-tissue interaction may stimulate angiogenic growth factors, with consequent neovascularization of the myocardium. These effects may lead to improvement in myocardial perfusion and reduction in anginal symptoms. The laser revascularization therapies of Transmyocardial and Percutaneous Myocardial Revascularization (TMR and PMR, respectively) are proposed as a means of ameliorating anginal symptoms, and neither technique has been purported to confer mortality benefit.

Patients with severe, chronic angina refractory to drug therapies, who are not suitable for traditional surgical or percutaneous revascularization approaches, may be candidates for the PMR™ technique. Suitable candidates include those with small target vessels, diffuse coronary disease, chronic total occlusions, and reversible myocardial ischemia.

The possibility of treatment by other revascularization techniques, such as coronary angioplasty or bypass graft surgery, should be explored. A site of reversible myocardial ischemia should be determined by nuclear or echocardiographic stress testing, to define a target area for laser channel creation. Echocardiographic assessment of left ventricular function and wall thickness in the target area are important, to avoid perforation of the ventricle during the procedure.

Contra-indications to laser PMR include significant aortic stenosis, peripheral vascular disease precluding a femoral approach, absence of reversible ischemic defect, thinned or scarred ventricular wall in the target area, left ventricular (LV) wall thickness of less than 8 mm, and poor left ventricular function, with a left ventricular ejection fraction (LVEF) of less than or equal to 30%, as measured by nuclear gated blood pool scan.

## Equipment

PMR™ is a percutaneous interventional cardiac procedure which must be done in an appropriately equipped cardiac catheterization laboratory. Medical, nursing, and technical staff should be cardiac catheterization laboratory trained and experienced in complex percutaneous cardiac interventions. The facility should also have the availability of "back up" surgery for acute complications, such as perforation and cardiac tamponade, which can arise as a result of the laser procedure.

The CardioGenesis PMR™ system (CardioGenesis Corporation, Sunnyvale, CA) comprises:

A single-use Axcis™ aligning or "guide" catheter:
The Axcis™ guide is a 9F braid-reinforced catheter with a soft distal tip and angulated end that allows the laser catheter to enter the left ventricle and be directed to the targeted area of myocardium. There are three guide shapes – Ultra 1, 2, and 3 – which differ according to the distance between the primary and secondary curves at the distal part of the catheter.

The Axcis™ laser catheter (Figure 8.1):
The Axcis™ laser catheter system is a 6F braid-strengthened shaft containing a central 400 μm optical fiber, fitted with a 1.75 mm lens mounted at the distal tip. The laser catheter is angulated at 90° distally, while at its proximal end the optical fiber has a fitting which allows connection to the laser source. The optical fiber with lens attachment can be independently advanced forwards from the outer sheath of the laser catheter (Figure 8.2).

The AdVent™ Holmium:yttrium-aluminum-garnet (Ho-YAG) laser:
The AdVent™ Ho:YAG laser is a portable self-contained system with a laser console and footswitch. The device weighs 350 lb (159 kg), produces a 632.8 nm laser beam for calibration, and 2 joule pulses ($\pm$ 10%) of infrared radiation at 5.7 kW peak power 83 J/cm$^2$ fluence and a wavelength of 2.1 μm, for treatment.

ECG monitoring system:
Internationally, the CardioGenesis PMR™ system, uses an ECG monitoring system that is microprocessor-controlled and generates a trigger signal synchronized with the R-waves of the subject's ECG. This allows a burst of two pulses of laser energy to be fired on depression of the footswitch, only when the R-wave trigger is sensed. A firing delay allows delivery of the laser energy, assuring contact of the fiber and lens with the endocardial surface during late systole, at the time of minimum ventricular movement and maximum wall thickness.

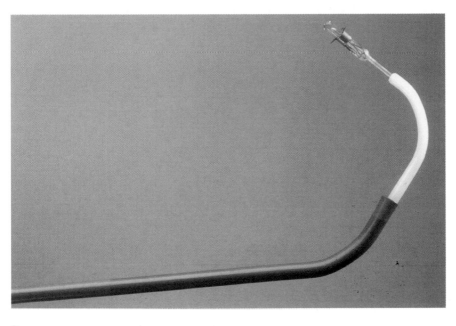

a

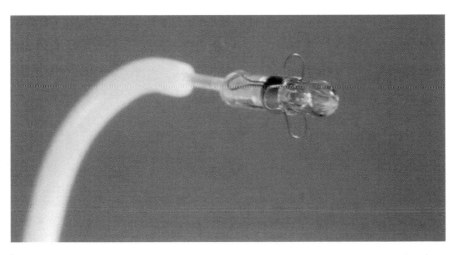

b

***Figure 8.1:*** *(a) The coaxial CardioGenesis<sup>TM</sup> laser system includes a 9F alignment catheter, a steerable laser fiber delivery catheter, and a 400 μm extendable optical fiber. (b) This close-up of the working end of the laser catheter reveals the petal array of nitinol wire that retards advancement of the activated laser catheter through the myocardium.*

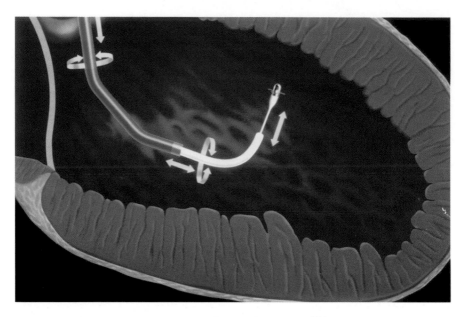

***Figure 8.2:*** *Schematic illustration of the CardioGenesis™ PMR system. Note the multiple degrees of rotational and longitudinal freedom that allow orthogonal access to all endocardial surfaces.*

## PMR technique using the CardioGenesis PMR™ system

There has been significant clinical experience using the CardioGenesis PMR™ system, with more than 300 human cases done worldwide, to date. The exact technique for the use of this device is as follows:

- Patients have routine cardiac catheterization laboratory preparation, and require little or no sedation for the percutaneous myocardial revascularization procedure. Vascular access is obtained by use of standard Seldinger technique. A 9F sheath is positioned in a femoral artery and venous access is obtained. Systemic anticoagulation is achieved using a bolus dose of heparin (5–8000 units) to attain a target ACT of about 250 s.
- A transparent film should be affixed on the screen of the catheter laboratory video monitor. A "roadmap" displaying the appropriate coronary distribution and outline of the ventricular cavity is to be marked on the transparent film. This "roadmap" assists in directing placement of the laser tip and creation of the channels in the target area.

- Selective coronary angiography is then done, with injection of the native coronary artery or bypass graft that best demonstrates the coronary anatomy in the targeted area. Demonstration of retrograde collaterals may also be required to define the source of blood flow to the area of interest. For example, the left anterior oblique-cranial view may allow the best definition of the myocardial surface of the left anterior descending-diagonal distribution, whereas the right anterior oblique-caudal view best defines the circumflex-marginal distribution. Orthogonal views should be recorded to allow later confirmation of the spatial orientation of the guide/laser catheter, and to verify adequate extension of the laser fiber and laser tip contact with the endocardial surface.

- The proximal and distal sidearm flush ports of the Axcis™ laser catheter system should each be connected to a 1 l bag of normal saline containing 2000 units heparin, which is placed in a pressure bag at 300 mmHg pressure. This allows for flushing of both the laser catheter and the aligning catheter.

- Using sterile technique, the proximal end of the Axcis™ laser catheter should then be connected to the output jack of the AdVent™ Ho:YAG laser. Calibration of the energy parameters is then done by placing the distal tip of the laser catheter inside the calibration "spool", which fits into the calibration port on the front of the laser console. Calibration is done within 60–120 s. The AdVent™ laser should then be switched to the "standby" mode, with the tip of the laser catheter removed from the spool. The apparatus is ready for use.

- The CardioGenesis PMR™ system guiding catheter is delivered retrograde across the aortic valve over a 125 cm, 6F pigtail catheter and a 0.035" J wire via the 9F femoral arterial access sheath. The guiding catheters have various preformed shapes (Ultra 1,2,3) that allow access to the endocardial surface for a diversity of left-ventricular contours. Once the pigtail catheter is passed across the aortic valve and positioned, left ventriculography is done with a standard power injector. The ventriculogram should be done in exactly the same optimal coronary angiographic and orthogonal views as described above.

- The 9F guide is positioned towards the apex of the left ventricular chamber, and, after removal of the pigtail catheter, the steerable laser delivery catheter should be advanced towards the tip of the guide. The laser delivery catheter carries the extendable optical fiber capped by a lens. The lens has a circular radio-opaque marker positioned 3 mm from the tip, which indicates the location and orientation of the laser fiber.

- As the laser fiber is advanced out of the guide catheter, the guide should be withdrawn using a "push and pull" maneuver, to avoid trapping the laser tip in the ventricular muscle.

**99**

- The guide and extendable laser delivery catheter are manipulated to direct the laser fiber to different sites in the target area. Independent rotation and advancement of the guide and laser delivery catheter allow for multiple degrees of freedom. The Axcis™ aligning guide is used for coarse positional adjustments, whilst movements of the inner delivery catheter and optical fiber are used for fine adjustments. Whenever the guide is moved along the longitudinal axis of the left ventricule, the central laser fiber should be withdrawn into the guide catheter.

- At fluoroscopy, when the radio-opaque marker appears circular, it is in a plane directly towards or away from the image intensifier. When in a plane directly perpendicular to the image intensifier, the marker appears as a solid bar. This marker also denotes the site of nitinol petals that extend perpendicular to the axis of the fiber and retard excessive advancement of the fiber when the laser is fired. The laser requires contact with the ventricular wall, so that a mild forward pressure should be applied during firing.

- At each channel site, contact should be confirmed by a view perpendicular to the axis of the catheter and the laser then activated. It is advisable to deliver a "burst" of two pulses of energy (2 J/pulse). Only one energy burst should be delivered at the apex, to avoid perforation of the left ventricle. In other target areas, the laser fiber should be advanced 1 mm after the first burst and a second burst then discharged, so that a total of 8 joules of energy is delivered to create each channel.

- Laser firing should occur in late systole, typically 100–150 ms after the QRS complex. As each channel is made, the position of the catheter tip should be marked on the "roadmap" transparency. Generally, 10–20 channels are made during the procedure, with the number being determined by the size of the target area and the spacing requirement of the channel per cm$^2$.

- Once all of the channels have been created, the guide and laser catheter apparatus are removed. The 6F pigtail catheter is then re-introduced into the left ventricle and a post-procedure LV-gram done to assess post-procedure LV function and regional wall motion. The newly created laser channels may be visible on ventriculography as short contrast-filled "spike-like" shafts radiating from the ventricular cavity.

- After the procedure, the patient is managed in a standard fashion, with bed rest and removal of the femoral sheaths when the ACT has dropped below 175 s. Patients are observed for 18–24 h, and generally can be discharged on the day following the PMR™ procedure.

- An echocardiogram is done routinely to document the presence or absence of pericardial effusion and to assess left ventricular and valve function. Other post-procedural tests include electrocardiogram, cardiac enzymes, serum urea, creatinine, and electrolytes.

**100**

- Follow-up has generally been with clinical review at 1 month, and, as part of the current clinical investigational protocol, exercise ECG and nuclear scans at 3 months and 6 months.

As for any cardiac surgery or percutaneous procedure, complications may occur as a consequence of the intervention. Complications specifically related to the laser revascularization procedure include development of ventricular arrhythmias, temporary bundle branch block, LV impairment, damage to heart structures, or perforation of the left ventricle or a coronary artery. In view of the small risk of cardiac tamponade, it is suggested that the laboratory have a transthoracic echocardiography machine and pericardiocentesis equipment readily available.

## Clinical studies

Since the first clinical reports of treatment, transmyocardial laser revascularization has been shown to significantly decrease Canadian Classification System (CCS) angina class at 3, 6, and 12 months, reduce perfusion defects in the treated free left ventricular wall in up to 76% of patients at 12 months, and reduce the number of admissions to hospital for angina.[1,2] Initial studies suggested that direct perfusion through patent channels may be the means by which laser revascularization techniques operate. However, more recent investigations implicate angiogenesis as the mechanism for the clinical effects of laser revascularization treatments.[3–5]

The initial feasibility study of percutaneous myocardial revascularization was done in a dog model using holmium:YAG laser energy delivered to the endocardial surface of the left ventricle via a femoral artery. Multiple channels could be created in anterior, lateral, inferoposterior and septal regions as shown by contrast ventriculography. Gross and histological examination confirmed channel sites and similarity of their appearance to laser channels created by the epicardial method of TMR.[6] Subsequently, a clinical study of the prototype device was undertaken in 30 patients with CCS class III-IV angina and disease not amenable to standard revascularization techniques. Results showed that clinical use of the PMR procedure was technically possible and safe.[7]

An early pilot study using the CardioGenesis PMR™ system reported safety with clinical application, a trend to reduction in CCS angina class from a mean of 3.4 to 1.6, and an improvement in total exercise treadmill duration from 300 s to 485 s (p = 0.01).[8]

The interim results of the PACIFIC trial, a prospective randomized trial comparing PMR™ plus medication with medication alone, reported a mean improvement in CCS angina class at 6 months of 1.4 versus 0.25 (p < 0.00001)

**101**

for the laser-treated group compared with the medication-alone group. In addition, there was up to 30% improvement in exercise duration at 6 months for the PMR treated group compared with an average 6% improvement for the medication-only group (p < 0.002). No significant increase in morbidity or mortality was reported between groups.[9] Longer term results are awaited.

The Pearl study, currently underway in Europe, is a randomized study to assess safety and efficacy of the CardioGenesis PMR™ system as a treatment for patients with stable angina who are not suitable for coronary bypass surgery or angioplasty. Recruitment should be completed by mid-1999.

New directions include development of the CardioGenesis™ system to enable delivery of angiogenesis factors at the time of PMR™. Such agents may include proteins, such as vascular endothelial growth factor (VEGF) or basic fibroblast growth factor (FGFI), which has been shown to stimulate angiogenesis in myocardial ischemia.[10] Alternatively, gene therapies, which code for local growth factor production, may also be delivered. The efficacy of combining laser PMR™ with growth factors to stimulate neovascularization requires further research.

## Conclusions

Percutaneous myocardial revascularization using the CardioGenesis PMR™ system uses energy from a holmium:YAG laser applied to the endocardial surface, through the use of a flexible, fiberoptic catheter conveyed via a guiding catheter from the femoral artery into the left ventricule. Delivered energy creates channels in the myocardium by vaporizing tissue in the targeted ischemic area. Initial studies of PMR™ have shown the feasibility and apparent safety of this method for clinical use. Early results of current randomized trials have reported significant improvements in duration of exercise and CCS angina class in patients with severe angina who are unsuitable for traditional revascularization therapies.

## References

1.  Mirhoseini M, Fisher J, Cayton M, Myocardial revascularization by laser: a clinical report. *Lasers Surg Med* 1983; **3**: 243–5.

2.  Horvath KA, Cohn LH, Cooley DA et al. Transmyocardial revascularization: results of a multicenter trial with transmyocardial laser revascularization used as sole therapy for end stage coronary artery disease. *J Thorac Cardiovasc Surg* 1997; **113**: 645–54.

3.  Cooley DA, Frazier OH, Kadipasaoglu KA et al. Transmyocardial revascularization: anatomic evidence of long-term channel patency. *Texas Heart Inst J* 1994; **21**: 220–4.

4. Kohmoto T, Fisher PE, DeRosa C et al. Evidence of angiogenesis in regions treated with transmyocardial laser revascularization. *Circulation* 1996; **94** (suppl II): 294.

5. Malekan R, Reynolds C, Narula N et al. Angiogenesis in transmyocardial laser revascularization: a nonspecific response to injury. *Circulation* 1998; **98** (suppl II): 62–5.

6. Kim CB, Kesten R, Javier M et al. Percutaneous method of laser transmyocardial revascularization. *Cathet Cardiovasc Diagn* 1997; **40:** 223–8.

7. Oesterle SN, Reifart NJ, Meier B et al. Initial results of laser-based percutaneous myocardial revascularization for angina pectoris. *Am J Cardiol* 1998; **82:** 659–62.

8. Lauer B, Junghans U, Stahl F et al. Percutaneous myocardial revascularization, a new approach to patients with intractable angina. *J Am Coll Cardiol* 1998; **31** (suppl A): 214A.

9. Oesterle SN, Yeung A, Ali N et al. The CardioGenesis percutaneous myocardial revascularization (PMR) randomized trial: initial clinical results. *J Am Coll Cardiol* 1999; **33** (suppl A): 380A (abstr).

10. Schumacher B, Pecher P, von Specht BU, Stegmann T. Induction of neoangiogenesis in ischemic myocardium by human growth factors: first clinical results of a new treatment of coronary heart disease. *Circulation* 1998; **97:** 645–50.

# 9. Excimer Laser Transmyocardial Revascularization System

Ramez EN Shehada, Thanassis Papaioannou and
Warren S Grundfest

## Introduction

Transmyocardial revascularization (TMR) has emerged as a promising treatment
for angina in ischemic heart disease patients who are not candidates for
angioplasty or coronary bypass surgery. The original laser-based technique
(TMLR) as proposed by Mirhoseini and colleagues[1,2] was developed to allow
direct perfusion from the ventricle into the myocardium, as in the reptilian heart.
Mirhoseini developed an EKG-triggered $CO_2$ laser to drill channels from the
epicardial to the endocardial surface. This laser was specially designed to drill a
TMR channel with single pulse, and Mirhoseini proposed that the channels
remained patent to perfuse the myocardium directly from the ventricle. Recent
research[3–6] has found that most of the channels close relatively quickly, which
suggests that the original hypothesis of direct perfusion from the ventricle is
incorrect and that TMLR may provide its benefits, if any, through other
mechanisms. The clinical advantages of the technique are evidenced by the
decreased intensity and frequency of angina, reduction in the need for antianginal
medications, and improved work capacity.[7–10] Despite multiple studies suggesting
clinical advantages, demonstration of improvement in cardiac function or survival
has been elusive. Various investigators have proposed the following hypotheses as
mechanisms of action of TMLR, although the observed clinical improvement may
result from a combination of some or all of these mechanisms.

- *Hypothesis 1*: Laser-drilled channels re-endothelialize, remain patent, and
  permit blood flow from the ventricle directly into the myocardium.[1,2,11]
- *Hypothesis 2*: Laser-drilled channels close, but as clot lysis occurs,
  interconnections are formed between various capillary beds (sinusoids).
  Release of growth factors, owing to cellular injury and the presence of
  platelets and thrombus in a confined space, induce angiogenesis, which
  increases vascular interconnections.[12–14]
- *Hypothesis 3*: Ablation and thermoacoustic destruction of some myocytes
  within a given myocardial volume allows redistribution of blood flow and
  improves oxygen supply to the surviving myocytes.[15]

- *Hypothesis 4*: Laser-drilled channels close, produce small scars and improve the compliance of the ventricle wall, allowing the heart to operate more efficiently.[16,17]
- *Hypothesis 5*: Laser-drilled channels and surrounding damage zones denervate the myocardium by injuring both pain and sympathetic nerves,[18] thereby reducing the anginal symptoms. Damaging the pain fibers reduces the perception of anginal pain, while the sympathectomy dilates the myocardial vessels to improve flow, which may reduce angina.
- *Hypothesis 6*: Laser-drilled channels change the conduction characteristics of ischemic myocardium and improve myocardial contractility and ventricular function (Dr Gerhard Muller, Berlin, Germany, personal communication).
- *Hypothesis 7*: Observed clinical improvement may bear no relation to the laser-drilled channels but may be a response to other factors, including optimization of and adherence to medication regimens, improved diet, appropriate rest and exercise, and placebo effects.

The initial choice of the short pulsed (50 ms) $CO_2$ laser was based on the desire to do the drilling before any significant myocardial motion, to create straight regular channels believed essential to maintain patency. In addition, the short pulse duration reduces thermal damage to the tissue surrounding the channel. Unfortunately, this large and cumbersome $CO_2$ laser has several inherent drawbacks for clinical use. First, the laser requires an articulated arm to deliver its energy, which precludes percutaneous catheter applications. Second, for safety, the laser can only be fired when the ventricle is filled with blood. Blood absorbs the laser energy after penetrating the endocardium, and prevents perforation of the posterior wall. The requirement of a full ventricle places constraints on application during surgery. Third, the laser can cut through the chordae tendineae to cause unsuspected mitral valve incompetence. The inability to regulate the deposition of laser energy precisely is a serious limitation of $CO_2$-based TMLR. Given the limitations of $CO_2$ laser-based TMLR, we investigated alternative energy sources that could be precisely controlled and produce minimal thermal damage.

Any effort to rationalize the choice of energy source for TMLR must be based on an understanding of how the channels produce the observed clinical benefits. However, since the mechanism of action of TMLR is currently unknown, the alternative is to choose an energy source based on a *hypothetical* mechanism or mechanisms of action, and to optimize the ablation process to produce the effects in the tissue. The inability to define the physiological basis for TMLR makes optimization difficult. For each of the above mechanisms, parameters can be chosen to produce specific tissue effects, such as denervation or hole drilling, with minimal thermal damage. Past experience with lasers in cardiovascular applications suggests that optimal clinical results are obtained by minimizing thermal and shock-wave injury to promote drilling without scarring. Thermal injury leads to intense collagen deposition and scarring. If producing small scars in the myocardial wall is the mechanism of action, then lasers are not required, since this can easily be accomplished using heated needles, ultrasound, or RF (radio frequency) current. The concept of denervating the myocardium to produce cardiac sympathectomy and to decrease the perception of anginal pain may provide clinical relief, but it may also have undesirable consequences, such as allowing overexertion leading to muscle damage. We assessed the performance of the XeCl excimer laser for TMLR, with emphasis on optimizing the channel-drilling parameters and minimum tissue damage. A series of in vivo experiments was done to identify the optimal delivery systems and laser settings that produce the most uniform tissue ablation with the least thermal and mechanical damage to the adjacent tissue.

# Materials and methods

## Laser and delivery system

A XeCl excimer laser (Model CVX 300, Spectranetics, Colorado Springs, CO, USA) operating at 308 nm was used. Laser pulses of 145 ns duration were delivered to the myocardium via a 1.4 mm diameter UV-grade multifiber (50 100 µm fibers) fiberoptic catheter (Spectranetics, Colorado Springs, CO). The latter was driven into the myocardium at preselected constant speeds by use of a computer-controlled mechanism (custom designed) shown in Figure 9.1. The actual handheld probe is shown in Figure 9.2. To determine the optimal channel-drilling settings, we varied the pulse repetition rate and the catheter advancement speed between 10–80 Hz and 0.1–15 mm/s, respectively. A constant fluence of 35 mJ/mm$^2$ was used throughout our experiments. This value has been previously determined, by in-vitro experiments in our laboratory, to be the optimal fluence for myocardial ablation.

## Animal model and experimental protocol

A total of 27 pigs weighing between 30–50 kg were used to model myocardial ablation in excimer-based TMLR. The animals were intubated and mechanically ventilated at 10 breaths/min with a tidal volume of 450 ml. Anaesthesia was induced by injecting thiopental into an ear vein, and was maintained by 1–2% isoflurane. The heart was exposed by either of two surgical approaches: a midline sternotomy or an intercostal incision between the third and fourth ribs. The pericardial sac was carefully opened to expose the anterior lateral wall of the heart. The TMR channels were opened through the myocardial wall of the left ventricle at different drilling settings. The animal was sacrificed 1 h after the

**107**

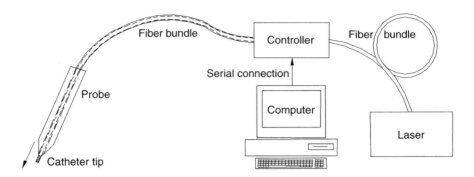

***Figure 9.1:*** *Computer-controlled electromechanical mechanism used to drive the optical-fiber catheter into the myocardium at preselected constant speeds.*

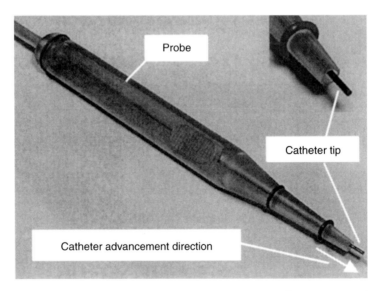

***Figure 9.2:*** *Actual handheld probe used to drive the multifiber optical catheter into the myocardium to drill the TMR channels.*

procedure, the heart was excised, and a section of myocardium surrounding each channel was dissected. Each section was placed in its own container for fixation in a 10% formalin solution for more than 48 h before embedding. The specimens were embedded in paraffin, stained with hematoxylin and eosin, and sectioned for light microscopy.

**108**

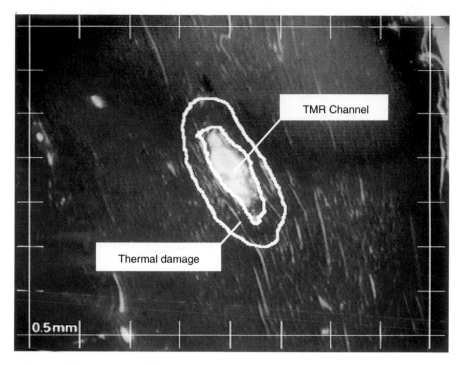

**Figure 9.3:** *Histology of a typical channel drilled in porcine myocardium using XeCl excimer laser, imaged under polarized light. The channel and a surrounding region of thermal damage are digitally outlined.*

## Histological analysis

Cross-sectional slides of the TMR channels were magnified by optical microscopy (Olympus BH-2 multiport at 12.5× or 40× objective lenses) and imaged under both normal and polarized light with a color video camera (Hitachi KP-C553 CCD, 722 × 492 pixels). Each image was digitized into 720 × 486 pixels with a frame grabber (Illuminator Pro CCIR-601, Matrox Electronics Inc, Dorval, Quebec, Canada). A digitizing pen tablet (Wacom SD420 E 12 × 12 digitizing tablet) was used to outline the channel periphery, which also represents the inner boundary of the thermally damaged region surrounding the channel. The outer boundary of this region was then outlined by marking the edge of the loss of birefringence. Increase in muscle temperature to above 60°C leads to a decrease in birefringence and hence a lower brightness when viewed with polarized light.[19,20] The assessment of changes in birefringence is an indicator of the extent of thermal injury.[19,20] Typical slide outlining is shown in Figure 9.3 of our results. The outlined digital images were analysed with specialized image processing

**109**

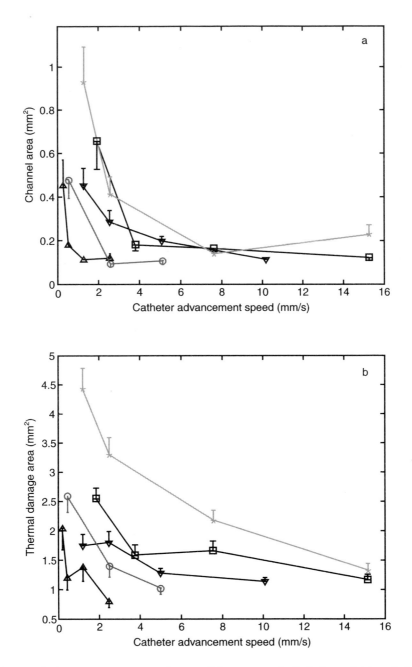

**Figure 9.4:** *Mean cross-sectional area of the excimer-drilled channel (a) and the thermal damage versus the catheter advancement speed (b) at pulse repetition rates of 10 (△), 20 (○), 40 (▽), 60 (□) and 80 Hz (*). Catheter diameter and fluence were 1.4 mm and 35 mJ/mm², respectively. Error bars represent one standard error of the mean (SEM).*

software (Matrox Inspector version 1.7, Matrox Electronic Systems Ltd) to determine the areas of the channel and thermal damage regions. A total of 515 tissue specimens were imaged and analysed.

## *Results*

The histology of a typical channel drilled in porcine myocardium with a XeCl excimer laser is shown in Figure 9.3, in which the channel and its surrounding region of thermal damage are digitally outlined. Histological analysis revealed wide variations in shape, size, and surrounding thermal damage of channels drilled at different catheter advancement speeds and pulse repetition rates. Channels drilled using the XeCl excimer laser showed changes in hole size and thermal damage zone in response to the lasing parameters.

The relation between the mean cross-sectional area of the channel and the catheter advancement speed at different pulse repetition rates is shown in Figure 9.4a. The mean area of the channel seems to depend on both catheter advancement speed and pulse repetition rate. The graphs indicate that the area of the channel tends to decrease almost exponentially with increasing catheter advancement speed. The decay rate of this exponential relation seems to decrease with increasing pulse repetition rate. In other words, the area of the channel becomes less sensitive to changes in the catheter advancement speed as the pulse repetition rate increases. Similarly, the extent of thermal damage decreases almost exponentially with increasing advancement speed and is also affected by the pulse repetition rate, as shown in Figure 9.4b. The area of thermal damage at any given advancement speed tends to increase with increasing pulse repetition rate.

The relation between channel-area increase and pulse repetition rate is shown in Figure 9.5a. The magnitude of this increase is dependent on the catheter advancement speed. At a given pulse repetition rate, slower catheter advancement speeds tend to produce larger channel areas, and vice versa. However, the channel area was insensitive to the doubling of the catheter advancement speed at a pulse repetition rate of 10 Hz. The dependency of the thermal damage area on the pulse repetition rate at different advancement speeds is shown in Figure 9.5b. At a constant advancement speed, the extent of thermal damage increases with rising pulse repetition rates, and vice versa. It is notable that within the pulse repetition range of 20–60 Hz, both the 1.27–2.54 mm/s advancement speeds appear to cause the same degree of thermal damage.

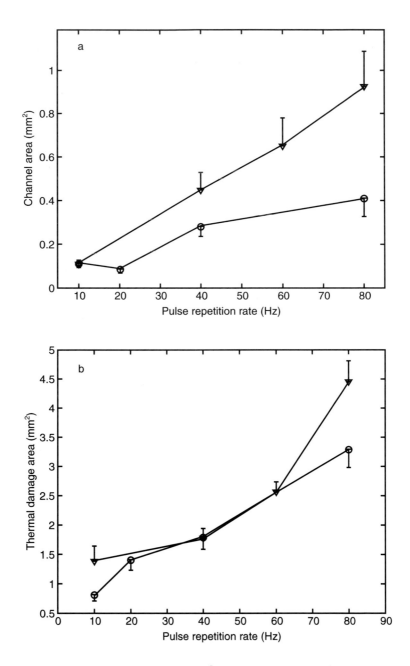

**Figure 9.5:** *Mean cross-sectional area of the channels (a) and their associated thermal damage zone (b) versus pulse repetition rate at a fluence of 35 mJ/mm², fiber diameter of 1.4 mm, and fiber advancement speed of 1.27 (▽) and 2.54 mm/s (○).*

# Discussion

We have assessed the performance of the XeCl excimer laser in drilling channels in the myocardium for TMLR. The excimer laser can operate over a broad range of repetition rates and energies that can be readily delivered via optical fibers. This flexibility requires assessment of several lasing parameters to determine those that give the optimal myocardial ablation for TMLR. The channels drilled by use of the XeCl excimer laser showed changes in the size of both the channel and thermal damage zone in response to the lasing parameters. These parameters are different from those commonly used for coronary artery recanalization. Of particular interest are the histological effects of the catheter advancement speed and the pulse repetition rate. Our results show that the catheter advancement speed is a crucial channel-drilling parameter. An increase in the advancement speed leads to a decrease in the size of both the channel and thermal damage for all repetition rates. For example, doubling the advancement speed from 1.27 to 2.54 mm/s leads to more than 50% decrease in the channel size for repetition rates of 20 Hz or more, as shown in Figure 9.5a. This suggests that at higher advancement speeds, the drilling process may be primarily due to mechanical tearing rather than ablation. The latter explanation is supported by histological evidence of increased tissue tearing and reduced thermal damage at higher speeds.

Advancement speeds slower than the laser ablation speed (= ablation rate × repetition rate) would increase the thermal damage mainly by deposition of subablative laser fluences. The ablation rate represents the tissue thickness ablated by each laser pulse, and it is dependent on both the fluence and type of tissue. On the other hand, advancement speeds that are faster than the laser ablation speed would increase tissue tearing, primarily by the impulsive pressure waves of the expanding ablation by-products confined in front of the catheter's tip. A good analogy of this process is the digging action of a pneumatic hammer. Higher advancement speeds will increase the pressure exerted by the catheter's tip on the tissue, and hence exaggerate the tearing impact of the pressure waves. Therefore, it is reasonable to assume that the optimal catheter advancement speed should be comparable or slightly faster than the laser ablation speed. Since the laser advancement speed is a function of the repetition rate, the value for optimal advancement speed would depend on the choice of repetition rate. For example, at an ablation rate of 40 μm/pulse and a pulse repetition rate of 40 Hz, the ablation speed is about 1.6 mm/s, and hence, the optimal advancement speed for this case should be around or slightly higher than the latter value. This way, the catheter tip will follow the ablation front, to produce the largest possible channel with minimal mechanical tearing. An advancement speed slightly slower than the ablation speed may also prove advantageous in displacing blood from the ablation site, thereby minimizing its interference with the ablation process.

**113**

Conversely, an advancement speed that is slightly higher than the ablation speed may prevent the accumulation of blood in the ablation site thus avoiding the strong shock waves generated by its ablation. Our results seem to suggest that slower advancement rates lead to larger holes but even larger thermal damage, while fast advancement rates lead to smaller holes with much less thermal damage. The physical basis of these effects needs to be investigated.

The histological results presented above could guide the process of optimizing excimer-based TMLR. The importance of our findings in the selection of lasing parameters in excimer-based TMLR can be shown by reviewing a recent study by Mack and colleagues.[14] Their study investigated the benefits of excimer-based TMLR over simple mechanical piercing achieved by driving the optical fiber into the myocardium without lasing. An output of 9 mJ, pulse repetition rate of 240 pulses/s, fiber advancement speed of 15.5 mm/s, and a fiber diameter of 600 μm were used for the TMLR procedure.[14] Our data show that those lasing parameters were not optimally matched for TMLR, and that their drilling effect is almost the same as mechanical piercing. A pulse repetition rate of 240 pulses/s and a fluence of 32 mJ produce an ablation speed of about 7.2 mm/s. This indicates that the fiber advancement speed should have been about 7.2 mm/s, instead of the 15.5 mm/s used in their study. At the latter advancement speed, the TMLR drilling was predominantly due to mechanical tearing by the advancing optical fiber.

The findings of our study have been used to develop an automated catheter advancement mechanism that exerts the minimal force required to keep the catheter's tip in contact with the myocardium and produce optimal ablation. The drive mechanism provides control on the ablation process and ensures operation at the optimal advancement speed.

## Conclusions

The histological measurements from our in vivo experiments indicate that XeCl excimer laser provides a precise method for creating TMR channels in the myocardium with minimal collateral tissue damage. The cross-sectional area of an excimer-drilled channel and the associated thermal damage are both increased with decreased catheter advancement speed for all pulse repetition rates. The optimal catheter advancement speed should be comparable or slightly faster than the ablation speed. Within the parameters tested, advancement speed of about 1.3 mm/s (~0.05"/s) and pulse repetition rates between 35–40 Hz appear to be optimal for excimer-based TMLR. While the mechanism of action of TMLR remains unknown, the 308 nm laser radiation offers a channel drilling technique compatible with either open-chest or percutaneous applications. The flexibility of the delivery system and the precise control of energy deposition afforded by ablation in the ultraviolet region (308 nm) could permit development of a safe percutaneous myocardial revascularization (PMR) technique.

## References

1. Mirhoseini M, Muckerheide M, Cayton MM. Transventricular revascularization by laser. *Lasers Surg Med* 1982; **2:** 187–98.

2. Mirhoseini M, Cayton MM, Shelgikar S, Fisher JC. Laser myocardial revascularization. *Lasers Surg Med* 1986; **6:** 459–61.

3. Krabatsch T, Schaper F, Leder C et al. Histological findings after transmyocardial laser revascularization. *J Card Surg* 1996; **11:** 326–31.

4. Whittaker P, Kloner RA, Przyklenk K. Laser-mediated transmural myocardial channels do not salvage acutely ischemic myocardium. *J Am Coll Cardiol* 1993; **22:** 302–9.

5. Kohmoto T, Fisher PE, Gu A et al. Does blood flow through holmium:YAG transmyocardial laser channels? *Ann Thorac Surg* 1996; **61:** 861–8.

6. Kohmoto T, Fisher PE, Gu A et al. Does blood flow through transmyocardial $CO_2$ laser channels? *J Am Coll Cardiol* 1996; 27 (suppl A): 13A (abstr).

7. Horvath KA, Cohn LH, Cooley DA et al. Transmyocardial laser revascularization: results of a multicenter trial with transmyocardial laser revascularization used as sole therapy for end-stage coronary artery disease. *J Thorac Cardiovasc Surg* 1997; **113:** 645–53.

8. Krabatsch T, Tambeur L, Lieback E et al. Transmyocardial laser revascularization in the treatment of end-stage coronary artery disease. *Ann Thoracic Cardiovasc Surg* 1998; **4:** 64–71.

9. Milano A, Pratali S, Tartarini G et al. Early results of transmyocardial revascularization with a holmium laser. *Ann Thorac Surg* 1998; **65:** 700–4.

10. Diegeler A, Schneider J, Lauer B et al. Transmyocardial laser revascularization using the Holmium-YAG laser for treatment of end stage coronary artery disease. *Eur J Cardiothorac Surg* 1998; **13:** 392–7.

11. Whittaker P, Rakusan K, Kloner RA. Transmural channels can protect ischemic tissue: assessment of long-term myocardial response to laser- and needle-made channels. *Circulation* 1996; **93:** 143–52.

12. Spanier T, Smith CR, Burkhoff D. Angiogenesis: a possible mechanism underlying the clinical benefits of transmyocardial laser revascularization. *J Clin Laser Med Surg* 1997; **15:** 269–73.

13. Pelletier MP, Giaid A, Sivaraman S et al. Angiogenesis and growth factor expression in a model of transmyocardial revascularization. *Ann Thorac Surg* 1998; **66:** 12-8.

14. Mack CA, Magovern CJ, Hahn RT et al. Channel patency and neovascularization after transmyocardial revascularization using an excimer laser: results and comparisons to nonlased channels. *Circulation* 1997; **96** (suppl): II-65–9.

15. Whitaker P, Kloner RA. Transmural channels as a source of blood flow to ischemic myocardium? Insights from the reptilian heart. *Circulation* 1997; **95:** 1357–9.

16. Horvath KA, Greene R, Belkind N et al. Left ventricular functional improvement after transmyocardial laser revascularization. *Ann Thorac Surg* 1998; **66:** 721–5.

17. Kadipasaoglu KA, Pehlivanoglu S, Conger JL et al. Long- and short-term effects of transmyocardial laser revascularization in acute myocardial ischemia. *Lasers Surg Med* 1997; **20:** 6–14.

18. Mueller XM, Tcvaearai HH, Genton CY et al. Transmyocardial laser revascularization in acutely ischemic myocardium. *Eur J Cardiothorac Surg* 1998; **13:** 170–5.

19. Whittaker P. Detection and assessment of laser-mediated injury in transmyocardial revascularization. *J Clin Laser Med Surg* 1997; **15:** 261–7.

20. Jansen ED, Frenz M, Kadipasaoglu KA et al. Laser-tissue interaction during transmyocardial laser revascularization. *Ann Thorac Surg* 1997; **63:** 640–7.

# II
# Therapeutic Myocardial Angiogenesis

# 10. Vascular Endothelial Growth Factor (VEGF) Protein Therapy for Ischemic Coronary Disease

Edward R McCluskey

## The VEGF molecule

Vascular endothelial growth factor (VEGF) is a vascular endothelial cell specific protein growth factor, which is necessary for angiogenesis during embryonic growth and is important in a number of physiological processes during adult life.[1] It is composed of two homodimeric subunits and contains both receptor and heparin binding domains. VEGF is produced by many different cell types in four isoforms. These isoforms have 121, 165, 189, and 206 amino acids in each of the homodimeric halves of the molecule. The 165 amino acid isoform of VEGF is distinctive in that it avidly binds heparin, which may be important in its use since the ability to bind heparan sulfate proteoglycans may allow localization of delivery.

VEGF has several biological activities. It is a potent angiogenic agent, and is able to stimulate blood vessel growth in a number of experimental models including the chick allantoic membrane, the rabbit cornea, the ischemic rabbit leg, and the ischemic pig myocardium. In addition to its angiogenic properties, VEGF can also cause vasodilation through the stimulation of the release of nitric oxide and can cause vascular permeability, reportedly through the actions of platelet activating factor and prostacyclin.[2] The latter two properties of vasodilation and vascular permeability were thought likely to constitute the dose limiting toxicity in preclinical experiments.

## VEGF for therapeutic angiogenesis

Several animal experiments have successfully shown the potential for VEGF-165 protein to act as a therapeutic angiogenesis agent. In 1994, Takeshita and colleagues[3] delivered VEGF-165 protein intra-arterially in a rabbit hindlimb ischemia model, and reported an increase in angiographically apparent new capillaries and an improvement in lower limb blood pressure. They referred to the procedure as "therapeutic angiogenesis" and speculated that it might prove a useful technique for treating patients with extensive vascular disease.

Therapeutic angiogenesis for cardiac ischemia was subsequently reported by several groups in different animal species. Banai and colleagues[4] reported an improvement in cardiac collateral blood flow and an increase in intramyocardial blood vessels in a dog model of cardiac ischemia after treatment with intracoronary VEGF-165 protein. They similarly speculated that exogenously administered VEGF might improve myocardial angiogenesis with resulting improved collateral blood flow. Similar findings were reported by Pearlman and colleagues[5] in a pig model of myocardial ischemia after treatment with VEGF-165 protein. That study reported an increase in myocardial collateralization and a resulting improvement in myocardial function after treatment with VEGF-165 protein. Subsequent studies have shown that VEGF-165 protein may be successfully used via several cardiac routes[6] and may even be effective in the pig model after intravenous administration.[7]

## Phase 1 clinical trials

Based on successful demonstrations of therapeutic angiogenesis in multiple animal models and on extensive toxicological safety and tolerability experience, Genentech Inc. began a program of clinical trials to test the principle of therapeutic angiogenesis in human beings by filing an Investigational New Drug application with the US FDA in November, 1997. The phase 1 trials described below were designed to test the safety and tolerability of different routes and rates of administration. If successful, these trials were to be followed by a phase 2 trial designed to investigate the efficacy of VEGF-165 in stimulating therapeutic angiogenesis. The phase 1 trials have now been successfully completed, and the phase 2 trial is currently underway.

The first phase 1A trial[8] was designed to determine if VEGF-165 protein could be safely and tolerably administered by intracoronary infusion to patients with severe coronary artery disease. Patients were eligible for participation if they had stable angina and areas of viable but underperfused myocardium (as shown by stress and rest nuclear perfusion scans). Since any risks or benefits were unknown, only patients who were not judged eligible for conventional revascularization (eg, PTCA, CABG) were included in the trial. Similarly, because of the unknown role of VEGF in diabetic retinopathy or in tumor angiogenesis, patients with diabetes or with any evidence of malignancy were excluded. Unstable angina, recent MI, CABG surgery, or ejection fraction of less than 25% were also exclusion criteria.

The trial was an open-label trial that studied a range of intracoronary infusion rates. A total of 15 patients were enrolled from six clinical centers: the Hennepin County Medical Center (Timothy D Henry); Prairie Education & Research Cooperative (Krishna Rocha-Singh); St. Elizabeth's Medical Center (Jeffrey

| Table 10.1  Criteria for "not tolerated" dose rate |
| --- |
| A:  Systolic blood pressure (SBP) change |
|      40 mm Hg if initial SBP > 160 |
|      30 mm Hg if initial SBP = 130 − 159 |
|      To <100 mm Hg if initial SBP < 130 |
| B:  Diastolic blood pressure change |
|      To <50 mm Hg |
|      To >100 mm Hg |
| C:  Heart rate |
|      To <50 with symptoms |
|      To <40 |
|      To >140 |
| D:  "Any clinical situation that, in the opinion of the investigator, has the potential to cause harm to the subject" |

Isner); The Christ Hospital (Dean Kereiakes); UC San Diego Medical Center (Frank Giordano); and Beth Israel Deaconess Medical Center (Michael Simons).

All patients received 20 min intracoronary infusion of VEGF-165 protein delivered at rates of 5, 17, 50, or 167 ng/kg/min. The primary goal of the study was to determine the tolerability of the infusion and a pre-specified set of criteria (Table 10.1) were outlined for calling a dose rate "not tolerated". There were to be four patients per group until one of the prespecified boundaries was crossed, at which point the trial would be concluded.

The three lowest infusion rates (5, 17, 50 ng/kg/min) were tolerated by all four patients per group. In the highest infusion-rate group (167 ng/kg/min), two or three patients did not tolerate the infusion and this rate was declared the "non-tolerated" rate, thus ending the trial.

In addition to determining the tolerability of the infusions, several other clinical parameters were also recorded at the beginning and end of the study. All patients underwent extensive physical and ophthalmological examination to assure the initial long-term safety of the VEGF infusions. Included in these assessments were treadmill times and the results of nuclear perfusion tests. Additionally, follow-up angiography was obtained for seven patients thought to have had improved nuclear perfusion studies. Although these additional data appeared promising with regard to showing therapeutic angiogenesis, no specific conclusions could be drawn from this open-label phase 1 study since no placebo group was included.

The phase 1B study[9] began after the successful conclusion of the phase 1A study. The goal of the phase 1B study was to determine the safety and tolerability of repeated intravenous administration of VEGF-165 protein.

Eligibility for the phase 1B study was very similar to the phase 1A study with the exception that patients with diabetes could be included in the phase 1B study if they met all other eligibility requirements, since all patients were examined by an ophthalmologist prior to enrollment and at the end of the study. A total of 28 patients were enrolled from seven centers: the Beth Israel Deaconess Medical Center (Michael Simons); UC San Diego Medical Center (Frank J Giordano); Hennepin County Medical Center (Timothy D Henry); UC Davis Medical Center (Gershony/Powell); Duke University Medical Center (Brian H Annex); University of Connecticut (Michael A Azrin); The Christ Hospital (Dean J Kereiakes).

In the phase 1B study, both the infusion rate and the total time of infusion were to be escalated (by group) during the study. In the first group of patients, VEGF-165 protein was intravenously administered for 1 h at a rate of 17 ng/kg/min on three separate occasions (days 1, 3, 7). Extensive blood sampling for VEGF immunoassay and pharmacokinetic analysis was done. In the first group, one patient had an allergic reaction (unknown whether it was to food, to VEGF, or to both), so a total of eight patients was studied. Since all patients in the lowest dose-rate group hemodynamically tolerated the infusion, the study proceeded to the next dose-rate group. At the 50 ng/kg/min rate, all four patients tolerated the 1 h infusion without difficulty. The next dose-rate group (100 ng/kg/min) was tolerated by only six of eight patients, and thus, by protocol, this dose rate was defined as the "non-tolerated" dose rate.

The next step in the protocol was to decrease the rate of infusion to the maximally tolerated rate (50 ng/kg/min) and to increase the length of time for each of the three infusions to 2 h and finally to 4 h. Four patients were enrolled in each of these last two groups and all tolerated the infusions without difficulties. Thus, the highest dose tolerated consisted of three intravenous infusions for 4 h each at an infusion rate of 50 ng/kg/min.

Throughout the study, extensive safety monitoring was done by physical examination and laboratory evaluations. No patient developed significant clinical changes thought to be due to VEGF administration and there were no changes in blood chemistry, hematological variables, or urinary variables. All patients underwent follow-up coronary angiography and ophthalmological examination. No patient showed angiographic progression of coronary artery disease and no patient showed abnormal ophthalmological changes. Promising changes were again seen in the other angiographic and nuclear variables but, again, without a control group, no valid conclusions could be drawn from these endpoints. The study concluded that VEGF-165 protein could safely be administered on multiple occasions by the intravenous route.

## Phase 2 clinical trials underway

Based on the successes of the phase 1 studies, a phase 2A study known as the VIVA study (VEGF in Ischemia for Vascular Angiogenesis) was begun in early 1998. This trial is a double-blind, placebo-controlled trial of the efficacy and safety of VEGF-165 protein in stimulating therapeutic angiogenesis in patients with coronary artery disease who are not optimally eligible for percutaneous or surgical revascularization by conventional means. To maximize the likelihood of a successful trial, patients were to be given VEGF on four occasions – a 20 min intracoronary infusion on day 0 followed by three intravenous infusions for 4 h on days 3, 6, and 9. Patients would be randomized to one of three groups – placebo, a "low-dose" group in which VEGF was to be infused (on all 4 occasions) at a rate of 17 ng/kg/min, and a "high-dose" group in which VEGF was to be infused at a rate of 50 ng/kg/min. The primary endpoint will be the change in exercise treadmill time at day 60. Additionally, changes in nuclear perfusion, angina class, and several quality of life indices will be studied. A subset of patients will undergo follow-up angiography to determine any visible evidence of angiogenesis. The preliminary results of that trial should be reported at the American College of Cardiology meeting in March, 1999, with complete analysis of the data later in the year.

## References

1. Ferrara N, Davis-Smyth T. The biology of vascular endothelial growth factor. *Endocr Rev* 1997; **18:** 4–25.

2. Murohara T, Horowitz JR, Silver M et al. Vascular endothelial growth factor/vascular permeability factor enhances vascular permeability via nitric oxide and prostacyclin. *Circulation* 1998; **97:** 99–107.

3. Takeshita S, Zheng LP, Brogi E et al. Therapeutic angiogenesis. A single intraarterial bolus of vascular endothelial growth factor augments revascularization in a rabbit ischemic hind limb model. *J Clin Invest* 1994; **93:** 662–70.

4. Banai S, Jaklitsch MT, Shou M et al. Angiogenic-induced enhancement of collateral blood flow to ischemic myocardium by vascular endothelial growth factor in dogs. *Circulation* 1994; **89:** 2183–9.

5. Pearlman JD, Hibberd MG, Chuang ML et al. Magnetic resonance mapping demonstrates benefits of VEGF-induced myocardial angiogenesis. *Nature Med* 1995; **1:** 1085–9.

**123**

6.  Lopez J, Laham R, Stamle A et al. VEGF administration in chronic myocardial ischemia in pigs. *Cardiovasc Res* 1998; **40:** 272–81.

7.  Giordano F, Ross JJ, Peterson K et al. Intravenous or intracoronary VEGF ameliorates chronic myocardial ischemia. *Circulation* 1998; **98:** I–455.

8.  Henry T, Rocha-Singh K, Isner J et al. Results of intracoronary recombinant human vascular endothelial growth factor (rhVEGF) administration trial. *Am Coll Cardiol* 1998; **31** (suppl A): 65A.

9.  McCluskey ER. VEGF protein for coronary disease. At: Clinical Angiogenesis: The Mini-Summit. Dallas, Texas: Cleveland Clinic Foundation, 1998.

# 11. Vascular Endothelial Growth Factor (VEGF) Gene Therapy for Peripheral and Coronary Artery Diseases

Douglas W Losordo, Peter R Vale and Jeffrey M Isner

## Summary

In patients in whom anti-anginal medications fail to provide sufficient relief from symptoms, additional interventions such as angioplasty or bypass surgery may be required. While both types of intervention are effective for various types of patients, many patients may not be candidates for either intervention owing to the diffuse nature of their coronary artery disease. Moreover, there are many patients in whom recurrent narrowing or occlusion of bypass conduits after initially successful surgery has left them with symptoms once more, but with no further angioplasty or surgical option. Ischemic muscle represents a promising target for gene therapy with naked plasmid DNA. Intramuscular (IM) transfection of genes encoding angiogenic cytokines, particularly those that are naturally secreted by intact cells, may be an alternative treatment strategy for patients with extensive tissue ischemia in whom contemporary therapies (anti-anginal medications, angioplasty, bypass surgery) have previously failed or are not feasible. This strategy is designed to promote the development of supplemental collateral blood vessels that will constitute endogenous bypass conduits around occluded native arteries – a strategy termed "therapeutic angiogenesis".

Preclinical animal studies from our laboratory have established that IM gene transfer may successfully accomplish therapeutic angiogenesis. More recently, phase 1 clinical studies from our institution have established that IM gene transfer may safely and successfully accomplish therapeutic angiogenesis in patients with critical limb ischemia. The notion that this concept could be extrapolated to the treatment of chronic myocardial ischemia was shown in our laboratory by administering recombinant human vascular endothelial growth factor (VEGF) to a porcine animal model of chronic myocardial ischemia. Recent experiments done in this same porcine model of myocardial ischemia have shown that direct intramyocardial gene transfer of naked plasmid DNA encoding VEGF (phVEGF$_{165}$, the identical plasmid used in our previous animal and human clinical trials) can be safely and successfully achieved via a minimally invasive chest-wall incision. Finally, initial results have supported the concept that intramyocardial injection of naked plasmid DNA encoding VEGF can achieve therapeutic angiogenesis as shown by clinical improvement in patients' symptoms and improved myocardial perfusion shown by SPECT-sestamibi imaging.

## Therapeutic angiogenesis as a new strategy for the treatment of ischemia

The therapeutic implications of angiogenic growth factors were identified by the pioneering work of Folkman and colleagues over two decades ago.[1] Their work documented the extent to which tumor development was dependent upon neovascularization, and suggested that this relation might involve angiogenic growth factors specific for neoplasms. Beginning a little over a decade ago,[2] a series of polypeptide growth factors were purified, sequenced, and shown to cause natural and pathological angiogenesis.

Subsequent investigations have established the feasibility of using recombinant formulations of such angiogenic growth factors to expedite and augment collateral artery development in animal models of myocardial and hindlimb ischemia. This new strategy for the treatment of vascular insufficiency has been termed "therapeutic angiogenesis".[3] The angiogenic growth factors first employed for this purpose were members of the FGF family. Baffour and colleagues[14] administered bFGF in daily intramuscular doses of 1 or 3 µg to rabbits with acute hindlimb ischemia; at the completion of 14 days of treatment, angiography and necropsy measurement of capillary density showed evidence of augmented collateral vessels in the lower limb, compared with controls. Pu and colleagues[5] used an acidic fibroblast growth factor (aFGF) to treat rabbits in which the acute effects of surgically induced hindlimb ischemia were allowed to subside for 10 days before beginning a 10-day course of daily 4 mg IM injections; at the completion of 30 days' follow-up, both angiographic and hemodynamic evidence of collateral development was superior to ischemic controls treated with IM saline. Yanagisawa-Miwa and colleagues[6] likewise showed the feasibility of bFGF for salvage of infarcted myocardium, but in that case growth factor was administered intra-arterially at the time of coronary occlusion, followed 6 h later by a second intra-arterial bolus.

We used the same animal model developed by Pu and colleagues[5] to investigate the therapeutic potential of a 45 kDa dimeric glycoprotein vascular endothelial growth factor (VEGF), isolated initially as a heparin-binding factor secreted from bovine pituitary folliculo-stellate cells.[7] VEGF was also purified independently as a tumor-secreted factor that induced vascular permeability by

**126**

the Miles assay,[8,9] and thus its alternate designation, vascular permeability factor (VPF). Two features distinguish VEGF from other heparin-binding angiogenic growth factors. First, the $NH_2$ terminus of VEGF is preceded by a typical signal sequence; therefore, unlike bFGF, VEGF can be secreted by intact cells.[10] Second, its high-affinity binding sites, which include the tyrosine kinase receptors *Flt-1*[11] and *Flk*/KDR,[12,13] are present on endothelial cells but not other cell types. Consequently, the mitogenic effects of VEGF – in contrast to acidic and basic FGF, both of which are mitogenic for smooth muscle cells,[14,15] fibroblasts, and endothelial cells – are limited to endothelial cells.[7,16] Interaction of VEGF with lower affinity binding sites has been shown to induce mononuclear phagocyte chemotaxis.[17,18]

VEGF has been shown to stimulate angiogenesis in vivo in experiments on rat and rabbit cornea,[19,20] the chorioallantoic membrane,[7] and the rabbit bone graft model.[20] We investigated the hypothesis that the angiogenic potential of VEGF was sufficient to constitute a therapeutic effect.[21] The soluble 165-amino acid isoform of VEGF ($VEGF_{165}$) was administered as a single intra-arterial bolus to the internal iliac artery of rabbits in which the ipsilateral femoral artery was excised to induce severe, unilateral hindlimb ischemia. Doses of 500–1000 μg of VEGF produced statistically significant augmentation of angiographically visible collateral vessels, and histologically identifiable capillaries. Consequent amelioration of the hemodynamic deficit in the ischemic limb was significantly greater in animals receiving VEGF than in non-treated controls (calf blood pressure ratio = $0.75 \pm 0.14$ *vs* $0.48 \pm 0.19$, $p < 0.05$). Serial angiography at baseline, and 10 and 30 days post-VEGF, disclosed progressive linear extension of the collateral artery of origin (stem artery) to the distal point of parent-vessel (re-entry artery) reconstitution in seven of nine VEGF-treated animals. Similar results were achieved in a separate series of experiments in which VEGF was administered by an intramuscular route daily for 10 days.[22] These findings were proof of principle for the concept that the angiogenic activity of VEGF is sufficiently potent to achieve therapeutic benefit.

Although each of these studies documented an increase in the number of angiographically visible collaterals, and increased capillary density in the muscles studied at necropsy, evidence regarding the physiological consequences of such anatomical improvement was limited to blood pressure measurements recorded in the ischemic versus the normal limb. Accordingly, we undertook a series of studies in the ischemic hindlimb model in which an intra-arterial Doppler wire,[23] sufficiently small (0.018 in) to measure phasic blood flow velocity in the rabbit's internal iliac artery, was used to investigate resting and maximum flow after therapeutic angiogenesis with a single, intra-arterial bolus of $VEGF_{165}$. By 30 days post-$VEGF_{165}$, flow at rest, as well as maximum flow velocity and maximum blood flow provoked by 2 mg papaverine, were all significantly higher in the VEGF-treated group.[24]

We further considered that one of the distinguishing features of VEGF mentioned above – the fact that the VEGF gene encodes a secretory signal sequence – might be exploited as part of a strategy designed to achieve therapeutic angiogenesis by arterial gene transfer. We had previously observed that site-specific transfection of rabbit ear arteries with the plasmid pXGH5 encoding the gene for human growth hormone (a secreted protein) yields local concentrations of human growth hormone equivalent to those of a physiological range, despite the fact that immunohistochemical examination of the transfected tissue disclosed evidence of successful transfection in less than 1% of cells in the transfected arterial segment.[25] Thus, gene products that are secreted may have profound biological effects, even when the number of transduced cells remains small. By contrast, for genes such as bFGF that do not encode a secretory signal sequence, transfection of a much larger cell population might be required for that intracellular gene product to express its biological effects.

We therefore applied 400 µg of phVEGF$_{165}$, encoding the 165-amino acid isoform of VEGF, to the hydrogel layer coating the outside of an angioplasty balloon,[26] and we delivered the balloon catheter percutaneously to the iliac artery of rabbits in which the femoral artery had been excised to cause hindlimb ischemia. Site-specific transfection of phVEGF$_{165}$ was confirmed by analysis of the transfected internal iliac arteries by reverse transcriptase-polymerase chain reaction (RT-PCR) and then sequencing the RT-PCR product. Augmented development of collateral vessels was shown by serial angiography in vivo, and increased capillary density at necropsy. Consequent amelioration of the hemodynamic deficit in the ischemic limb was shown by improvement in the calf blood pressure ratio (ischemic/normal limb) to $0.70 \pm 0.08$ in the VEGF-transfected group versus $0.50 \pm 0.18$ in controls ($p < 0.05$). Angiographic and histological evidence of angiogenesis were subsequently shown after intra-arterial gene transfer of phVEGF$_{165}$ in a human patient.[27] These findings thus established that site-specific gene *transfer* can be used to achieve physiologically meaningful *therapeutic* modulation of vascular disorders, including therapeutic angiogenesis. Of note, neither our intra-arterial animal studies nor our human clinical experience have disclosed any evidence of immunological toxicity.

## *Gene transfer of cDNA encoding for secreted protein may result in meaningful biological outcomes despite low transfection efficiency*

In experiments that have relied exclusively on the use of non-secreted gene products, examination by histochemical staining, in situ hybridization, and polymerase chain reaction has suggested that the transfection efficacy of direct gene transfer to vascular smooth muscle cells within the arterial wall was considerably less than 1% and might therefore preclude a meaningful biological response. By contrast, genes encoding for a secreted protein may overcome the handicap of inefficient transfection by a paracrine effect, secreting adequate protein to achieve local concentrations that may be physiologically meaningful. Nabel and colleagues[28] showed that despite similarly low efficiencies, cell surface protein expression resulting from percutaneous transfection of vascular smooth muscle cells with the histocompatibility gene HLA-B7 may be adequate to induce a biological response (focal vasculitis). Necropsy evidence of a pathobiological response after arterial gene transfer was reported by the same group in the case of transgenes encoding for the secreted proteins PDGF-B[29] and FGF-1;[30] in the former study, only 0.1 to 1% of cells in the artery segment were estimated to contain plasmid DNA by PCR approximation.

To determine more specifically the relation between a secreted gene product and transfection efficiency after in vivo arterial gene transfer, we devised in vitro[31] and in vivo[25] models to serially monitor expression of a gene encoding for a secreted protein. In vivo analyses were done on the central artery of the rabbit ear. Liposome-mediated transfection of plasmid DNA containing the gene for human growth hormone (hGH) was successful in 18 of 23 arteries. Serum hGH concentrations measured 5 days after transfection ranged from 0.1 to 3.8 ng/ml (mean 0.97 ng/ml); by contrast, serum drawn from the control arteries showed no evidence of hGH production. Serial measurement of hGH from transfected arteries showed maximum hGH secretion 5 days after transfection and no detectable hormone after 20 days. Despite these concentrations of secreted gene product documented in vivo, immunohistochemical staining of sections taken from the rabbit ear artery at necropsy disclosed evidence of successful transfection in less than 0.1% of cells in the transfected segment. Thus, low-efficiency transfection with a gene encoding for a *secreted* protein may achieve therapeutic effects not realized by transfection with genes encoding for proteins that remain intracellular.

We infer that this principle – in combination with the fact that ischemic skeletal muscle itself serves to augment transfection efficacy[32,33] – similarly accounts for the bioactivity that we have observed after gene transfer of naked DNA by direct injection into skeletal muscle.

## *Preclinical animal studies have established that intramuscular gene transfer may successfully achieve therapeutic angiogenesis*

Ten days after ischemia was induced in one hindlimb of New Zealand White rabbits, 500 μg of phVEGF$_{165}$ or the reporter gene LacZ were injected into the ischemic hindlimb muscles. Site-specific transgene expression was documented by mRNA and immunohistochemistry. At 30-day follow-up, angiographically recognizable collateral vessels and histologically identifiable capillaries were increased in VEGF-transfectants compared with controls. This augmented vascularity improved perfusion to the ischemic limb, as shown by a superior calf blood pressure ratio for $phVEGF_{165}$ ($0.84 \pm 0.09$) versus controls ($0.67 \pm 0.06$, $p < 0.01$); by improved blood flow in the ischemic limb (measured using an intra-arterial Doppler wire) at rest ($phVEGF_{165} = 22.7 \pm 4.6$, control $= 14.9 \pm 1.7$ ml/min, $p < 0.01$) and following a vasodilator ($phVEGF_{165} = 52.5 \pm 12.6$, control $= 38.4 \pm 4.3$, $p < 0.05$); and by increased distribution of labeled microspheres to the adductor muscle ($phVEGF_{165} = 4.3 \pm 0.5$, control $= 2.9 \pm 0.6$ ml/min/100 g tissue, $p < 0.05$), as well as the gastrocnemius muscle ($phVEGF_{165} = 3.9 \pm 0.8$, control $= 2.8 \pm 0.9$ ml/min/100 g tissue, $p < 0.05$) of the ischemic limb). A more detailed description of this study has been published previously.[32]

Ischemic muscle thus represents a promising target for gene therapy with naked plasmid DNA. IM transfection of genes encoding angiogenic cytokines, particularly those that are naturally secreted by intact cells, may constitute an alternative treatment strategy for patients with extensive tissue ischemia, in whom contemporary revascularization (anti-anginal medications, angioplasty, bypass surgery) have previously failed or are not feasible.

## Phase 1 clinical studies have established that intramuscular gene transfer may successfully achieve therapeutic angiogenesis

Gene transfer was done in ten limbs of nine patients with non-healing ischemic ulcers ($n = 7$) and/or rest pain ($n = 10$) due to peripheral arterial disease. A total of 4000 µg naked plasmid DNA encoding the secreted 165-amino acid isoform of human VEGF ($phVEGF_{165}$) was injected into ischemic muscles of the affected limb. Mean follow-up at the time of this submission was $6 \pm 3$ months (range 2 to 11 months). Local intramuscular gene transfer induced no or mild local discomfort up to 72 h after the injection. Serial CPK measurements remained in the normal range and there were no signs of systemic or local inflammatory reactions. To date, no aggravated deterioration in eyesight due to diabetic retinopathy or growth of latent neoplasm has been recorded in any patient treated with $phVEGF_{165}$ gene transfer. The only complication observed in the trial was limited to transient lower extremity oedema, consistent with VEGF-enhancement of vascular permeability.

**130**

## Transgene expression

Blood concentrations of VEGF transiently peaked 1–3 weeks after gene transfer in seven patients amenable to weekly assays. In two patients, baseline and/or more than two follow-up blood samples were not achievable. Clinical evidence of VEGF (vascular permeability factor) overexpression was evident by the observation of peripheral oedema development ($+1$ to $+4$ by gross inspection) in the six patients with ischemic ulcers. In four patients, the oedema was limited to the treated limb, while in two patients the contralateral limb was affected as well, albeit less severely. Oedema corresponded temporally to the rise in serum VEGF concentrations

## Noninvasive arterial testing

The absolute systolic ankle or toe pressure increased in nine limbs after gene transfer and was unchanged in one limb at the time of the most recent follow-up ($p = 0.008$). The ABI and/or TBI increased from $0.33 \pm 0.05$ (range $= 0$ to $0.58$, $n = 10$) at baseline to $0.43 \pm 0.04$ ($0.22$ to $0.57$, $p = 0.028$, $n = 10$) at 4 weeks; to $0.45 \pm 0.04$ ($0.27$ to $0.59$, $p = 0.016$, $n = 10$) at 8 weeks; and to $0.48 \pm 0.03$ ($0.27$ to $0.67$, $p = 0.017$, $n = 8$) at 12 weeks. Improvement in the pressure index was sustained, but did not rise significantly further after the second gene transfer.

Exercise performance improved in all five patients with rest pain or minor ischemic ulcers who underwent a graded treadmill exercise. All patients had a significant increase in pain-free walking time ($2.5 \pm 1.1$ min before gene therapy *vs* $3.8 \pm 1.5$ min at an average of 13 weeks after gene therapy, $p = 0.043$) and absolute, claudication-limited walking time ($4.2 \pm 2.1$ min *vs* $6.7 \pm 2.9$ min, $p = 0.018$). Two patients reached the target endpoint of 10 minutes of exercise.

## Angiography

Digital subtraction angiography showed newly visible collateral vessels at the knee, calf, and ankle levels in six of ten ischemic limbs treated. The luminal diameter of the newly visible vessels ranged from 200 μm to more than 800 μm, although most were closer to 200 μm and these frequently appeared as a "blush" of innumerable collaterals. Collaterals did not regress on follow-up angiography. Magnetic resonance angiography showed qualitative evidence of improved distal flow with enhancement of signal intensity, as well as an increase in the number of newly visible collaterals in eight limbs.

## Change in limb status and ischemic rest pain

Therapeutic benefit was shown by regression of rest pain, improved limb integrity, or both. The frequency of ischemic rest pain expressed as afflicted nights per week decreased significantly (5.9 ± 2.1 at baseline *vs* 1.5 ± 2.8 at 8 weeks' follow-up, p = 0.043), with a slight reduction of analgesic medication (on average from 1.8 to 1,5 analgesics/24 h). Based on criteria proposed by Rutherford, limb status improved in nine of ten extremities treated. Moderate improvement, including *both* an upward shift in the clinical category (at least one clinical category in patients with rest pain and at least two categories to reach the level of claudication in patients with tissue loss) and an increase in the ABI of more than 0.1 was documented in five cases. In one patient, an ischemic ulcer resolved sufficiently to allow placement of a split-thickness skin grafting, leading to absolute limb salvage. In two patients in whom a major amputation would have been inevitable, retention of a functional foot by a minor (toe) amputation was reached. Minimal improvement, including an upward shift in clinical category *or* improvement of the ABI of more than 0.1 occurred in another three cases. However, in two patients with an extensive forefoot necrosis and osteomyelitis, a below-knee amputation was required despite significant hemodynamic and angiographic improvement. There was one patient with progressive toe gangrene, who remained unchanged from his hemodynamic and angiographic findings. The patients underwent a below-knee amputation 8 weeks after gene therapy.

**Immunohistochemistry and molecular analysis**

Tissue specimens derived from one amputee 10 weeks after gene therapy showed foci of proliferating endothelial cells. This finding was particularly striking given an estimated endothelial cell turnover of "thousands of days" in quiescent microvasculature. PCR done on these samples showed persistence and widespread distribution of DNA fragments unique to $phVEGF_{165}$. Noteworthy amplification of DNA fragments was shown in muscle and skin samples derived from the site of injection, as well as in several muscle samples remote from the site of injection. Southern blot analysis confirmed persistance of intact plasmid DNA in muscle specimen derived from two amputeess 8 and 10 weeks after gene therapy. These findings are described in more detail in *Circulation*.

# Administration of human recombinant VEGF protein to a porcine model of myocardial ischemia augments myocardial collateral vessel development and improves myocardial perfusion

The treatment of ischemic heart disease is aimed at maintenance of a positive balance between oxygen supply and oxygen demand in the myocardium. The first choice for therapy in many patients will be pharmacological therapy. However, in those patients in whom anti-anginal medications fail to provide sufficient relief from symptoms, additional interventions such as angioplasty or bypass surgery may be required. While both types of intervention have been shown to be effective for various types of patients, many patients may not be candidates for either intervention due to the diffuse nature of their coronary artery disease. Moreover, there are many patients in whom recurrent narrowing or occlusion of bypass conduits after initially successful surgery has left the patient with symptoms once more, but with no further angioplasty or surgical option.

To test the efficacy of therapeutic angiogenesis for chronic myocardial ischemia, 18 Yorkshire pigs underwent a left thoracotomy followed by placement of an ameroid constrictor around the proximal circumflex coronary artery. Gradual occlusion of the artery ($26 \pm 4$ days) was accompanied by identifiable hypokinesis of the posterolateral wall of the left ventricle (2D echo). 30 days afterwards, recombinant human (rh) $VEGF_{165}$ protein (2 mg: $n = 8$) or saline ($n = 10$) was administered directly into the left coronary ostium. Post-adenosine myocardial perfusion studies that used colored microspheres 30 days later showed superior blood flow in the ischemic zone of the rhVEGF treated hearts (ischemic/normal ratio 1.09 $vs$ 0.97, $p < 0.05$) compared with those receiving saline injection. Four of eight rhVEGF treated animals succumbed to severe hypotension after rhVEGF administration. Therefore, 500 μg of rhVEGF was administered intracoronary to five normal pigs. A significant drop in mean arterial pressure ($-44.4 \pm 3.2\%$, $p < 0.05$ $vs$ baseline) and peripheral resistance ($-13.2 \pm 4.5\%$, $p < 0.05$ $vs$ baseline) was accompanied by increased heart rate. Intravenous administration of $N^{\omega}$-nitro-L-arginine (L-NNA), an inhibitor of nitric oxide (NO) synthase, restored blood pressure to baseline.

Thus, a single intra-coronary bolus of recombinant human VEGF protein is capable of significantly augmenting flow to collateral-dependent ischemic myocardium. Administration of rhVEGF protein, however, was complicated by hypotension, apparently mediated by VEGF-induced release of NO. These findings are summarized in the *Journal of Surgical Research*.

## *Intramyocardial gene transfer can be safely and successfully achieved via a minimal invasive chest-wall incision*

Given that the experiments described above established that VEGF could augment myocardial angiogenesis, we next sought to establish the safety of intramyocardial gene transfer by direct intramuscular injection. Previous experiments in our laboratory[34] had shown that this could be achieved in smaller animal models. Therefore, we undertook direct intramyocardial injection of both plasmid DNA encoding the reporter gene β-galactosidase, as well as a plasmid encoding $VEGF_{165}$ ($phVEGF_{165}$).

## Plasmids used

A nuclear-specific naked DNA encoding for β-galactosidase transcriptionally regulated by the CMV promoter/enhancer (pCMVβ) was used to assess the appropriate injection volume for intramyocardial injection.

## Animal model

A total of 23 Yorkshire pigs weighing 23–35 kg were studied. Animals were given a normal diet. All procedures were done under anesthesia. A 6F left Judkins coronary diagnostic catheter was advanced via the arterial introducer sheath to the ostium of the left coronary artery. After injection of 500 μg nitroglycerin into the left main coronary artery, cine-angiography was recorded in the 30° left anterior oblique position. Angiography was repeated from the same angles at follow-up just before sacrifice.

## Histological assessment

The heart of each animal was removed, examined for gross pathological changes, weighed, and rinsed in cold phosphate-buffered saline (PBS). The left ventricle was then dissected free and sliced transversally, perpendicular to the long axis of the heart, into slices 1 cm thick at five different levels from apex to the base of the heart. From each slice, sections were taken from anterior, lateral, posterior, and septal regions. Sections stained with hematoxylin and eosin were used to assess the extent of inflammatory infiltrates, and myocyte necrosis and fibrosis. In addition, biopsies from right ventricle, right atrium, left atrium, lung, liver, mediastinal lymph nodes, and pericardium were similarly assessed.

## Assessment of gene expression

In the pigs injected with pCMVβ, β-galactosidase activity in the myocardial tissue was assessed with a chemoluminescence assay (Tropix). Before measuring β-galactosidase activity, tissue homogenates were pretreated with Chelex 100 to inactivate a natural inhibitor of the enzyme.[35] In the pigs in which myocardium was injected with $phVEGF_{165}$, gene expression was assessed with SDS-PAGE western blotting for VEGF-protein as described elsewhere.[36] Tissue specimens were stored at 80° until assayed. The tissue was homogenized in lysis buffer, and spun down twice at high speed. Equal amounts (100 μg) of protein were loaded on a 12% gel under reducing conditions. After blotting, the membrane was exposed to a rabbit anti-VEGF antibody (Santa-Cruz sc152), followed by the secondary (anti-rabbit) antibody labeled with horseradish peroxidase. Finally the membrane was put into ECL solution and exposed to x-ray film.

## Results

Intramyocardial injections caused no changes in heart rate (pre-injection $138 \pm 12$ beats/min *vs* post-injection $142 \pm 10$), systolic blood pressure ($87 \pm 12$ *vs* $86 \pm 11$ mmHg) or diastolic blood pressure ($53 \pm 12$ *vs* $50 \pm 10$ mmHg). During injection, ventricular arrhythmias were rare. In one pig, non-sustained ventricular tachycardia (VT) without hemodynamic deterioration occurred during injection. In the remaining pigs, sporadic premature ventricular contractions (PVCs) occurred at the moment the needle entered the myocardium. No additional arrhythmias occurred in these pigs.

Online ultrasound monitoring showed that the administered plasmid DNA was distributed several cm beyond the site of needle entry.

Electrocardiography did not show evidence of myocardial infarction in any pigs. Creatine phosphokinase (CPK) concentrations increased from $457 \pm 233$ at the beginning of the procedure to $727 \pm 212$ at the end of the procedure, and to $4741 \pm 4035$ IU/l after 1 day. The myocardial specific MB isoenzyme, however, did not increase ($1.7 \pm 0.5$; $2.0 \pm 0.7$; $3.2 \pm 2.0$ mg/ml). None of the pigs had an MB fraction higher than the normal limit (5.0 ng/ml).

Among the pigs sacrificed after 1 week, left ventricular ejection fraction (LVEF) was unaffected by the volume of injectates: specifically, LVEF remained about 30% whether 4.5 ml, $4 \times 2.0$ ml, or $4 \times 5$ ml were used. Moreover, there was no statistically significant alteration in LVEF at any follow-up time compared with baseline. After 8 weeks, LVEF was $39 \pm 8\%$. Echocardiography disclosed no regional wall motion abnormalities in pigs studied 1 week (n = 2), 4 weeks (n = 3), or 8 weeks (n = 2) after treatment.

Histological examination of 276 sections retrieved at necropsy from 12 pigs disclosed only occasional foci of mononuclear inflammatory cells, typically less than four per high power field (HPF). Most (>90%) HPFs included no inflammatory cells. Foci of necrosis or fibrosis were limited to myocardium subserved by the occluded artery in the porcine model of myocardial ischemia. Histological examination of sections retrieved from all non-cardiac sites showed no evidence of pathological findings.

Plasma samples from the treated pigs were drawn before treatment and after treatment. Samples were drawn daily during the first week, and after 1 and 2 weeks where appropriate.

Furthermore, tissue specimens from different levels in the heart were taken at the end of the follow-up period to investigate local production of VEGF protein

**135**

by western blotting. In the pigs with a short follow-up, strong VEGF bands were present, typically showing a gradient with the strongest band closest to the injection site. At the end of the 4 weeks follow-up, either no or very vague VEGF bands were present for the lateral (Lat), anterior (ant), and posterior (post) part of the left ventricle.

Finally, among pigs with the occlusion of the left circumflex coronary artery induced by an ameroid constrictor diagnostic angiography typically showed enhanced filling (Rentrop score 3–4) of the left obtuse marginal branch (LOM) of the left circumflex coronary artery, reconstituted by one or more collateral vessels from the left anterior descending (LAD) or diagonal branches of the LAD coronary artery.

## Gene therapy for myocardial angiogenesis: initial clinical results with direct intramyocardial injection of phVEGF$_{165}$ as sole therapy for myocardial ischemia

This report describes the initial clinical experience with myocardial gene transfer as sole therapy for refractory angina pectoris. Patients were enrolled in the previously approved IND study. 16 patients with chronic, severe angina underwent direct intramyocardial gene transfer of naked DNA encoding vascular endothelial growth factor (VEGF). There were no operative complications. There was one late death (136 days). All patients had marked improvement in symptoms, objective evidence of improved myocardial perfusion, or both. This preliminary clinical experience suggests that therapeutic angiogenesis is a potentially useful strategy for patients with end-stage coronary artery disease.

### Patients

Patients were eligible for intramyocardial gene therapy if they had stable exertional angina (functional class 3 or 4) not in a setting of life-threatening ischemia and that was refractory to maximum medical therapy; areas of viable but underperfused myocardium on stress SPECT myocardial perfusion study; and multivessel occlusive coronary artery disease, occlusion of one or more coronary artery bypass grafts, or both. All patients meeting these criteria had to have a document of referral from their physician stating that the patient was refractory to medical therapy and was not a candidate for percutaneous or surgical revascularization. Upon receiving the document, an eligibility review committee comprised of three physicians (all unassociated with the investigation, two of whom were unassociated with SEMC), was required to provide unanimous agreement that the patient was an appropriate candidate for myocardial gene therapy.

Patients were excluded from enrollment if they had: successful coronary artery bypass graft (CABG) surgery, angioplasty, or myocardial laser revascularization in the 6 months before study screening; evidence of cancer; fundoscopic signs of diabetic retinopathy or age-related macular degeneration; or left ventricular ejection fraction of less than 20%.

All patients continued their routine medical therapy as needed after gene therapy.

## Plasmid DNA (phVEGF$_{165}$)

All patients received a eukaryotic expression vector encoding the 165-aminoacid isoform of the human VEGF gene[10,37] transcriptionally regulated by the cytomegalovirus promoter/enhancer (phVEGF$_{165}$).[27,38] Preparation and purification of the plasmid from cultures of phVEGF$_{165}$-transformed *E coli* were done in the SEMC Human Gene Therapy Laboratory by use of the column method (Qiagen Mega Kit). The purified plasmid was stored in vials and pooled for quality control analysis.

## Intramyocardial phVEGF$_{165}$ transfer

Plasmid DNA (125 µg) was reconstituted in sterile saline at room temperature and administered by direct intramyocardial injection in 4 aliquots of 2.0 ml each. All four injections were done via a "mini-thoractomy" either through the bed of the fifth costal cartilage or the fifth intercostal space, allowing access to the anterior, lateral, and apical portions of the left ventricle (LV) and to the interventricular septum. A stabilizing device (CardioThoracic Systems, Cupertino, CA) usually used to ensure vascular anastomosis during beating heart bypass, was used to ensure an immobile field for intramyocardial injection. Injection sites were selected according to the areas of ischemia identified by sestamibi imaging. Continuous transesophageal echocardiographic monitoring was done throughout the procedure to monitor development of wall motion abnormalities associated with injection of plasmid, and to ensure that plasmid DNA was not injected into the LV cavity. After completing the injections the pericardium was left partially open, a chest tube was inserted into the left pleural space, and the thoractomy incision was closed. Patients were extubated in the operating room and monitored post-operatively in intensive care according to the protocol used for minimally invasive CABG.

## SPECT myocardial perfusion study

Patients underwent a dobutamine SPECT-sestamibi study with dobutamine infusion up to 40 µg/kg/min. The acquisition of the post-stress SPECT image

**137**

began 10 min after the end of the stress period. Redistribution images were recorded either before or at least 4 h after stress with the patient at rest. Redistribution and reinjection data were reconstructed in short-axis, vertical, and longitudinal long-axis views for analysis. Using the 13-segment model, viability and perfusion scores were assigned to each segment based on the results of the nuclear scan. Perfusion was recorded as normal or abnormal. Segments were visually characterized as fixed, partially reversible, or totally reversible. On days 30 and 60, patients underwent repeat nuclear perfusion testing by use of the identical stress protocol and isotope used at baseline.

## Coronary angiography

Patients underwent diagnostic angiography less than 1 month before and 60 days after gene transfer. All angiograms were interpreted by a reviewer unaware of the patient's name, date of study, and sequence of study (ie, pre- vs post-treatment). A so-called collateral score was established for each film using the classification proposed by Rentrop and colleagues.[39] In short, collaterals were graded as absent (0), filling of side-branches of a target occluded epicardial coronary artery via collaterals without visualization of the epicardial coronary artery itself (1+), partial filling of the epicardial segment via collateral arteries (2+), or complete filling of the epicardial segment (3+). Each pair of films (baseline and follow-up) was scored independently.

## Statistical analysis

Data were reported as mean $\pm$ SEM. Comparisons between paired variables were made by Students $t$ test at a significant level of $p < 0.05$.

# Results

## Perioperative course

All patients underwent successful myocardial gene transfer. Mean operative time was 77 $\pm$ 6 min. Patients were extubated 34 $\pm$ 4 min postoperatively. Injections caused no changes in heart rate (60 $\pm$ 15/min vs 66 $\pm$ 16 /min), systolic blood pressure (120 $\pm$ 20 mmHg vs 132 $\pm$ 17 mmHg), or diastolic blood pressure (60 $\pm$ 5 mmHg vs 69 $\pm$ 5 mmHg). Ventricular arrhythmias were limited to unifocal extrasystolic beats (maximum n = 5) at the moment of injection. CO did not change significantly (pre-GA 4.8 $\pm$ 1.4 vs post-GA 4.4 $\pm$ 1.3 vs 24 h 4.3 $\pm$ 1.4, p = NS). Serial ECGs showed no evidence of myocardial infarction in any patient. Intraoperative blood loss was 0–50 cm$^3$ and total chest tube drainage was 30–395 cm$^3$. There were no major perioperative complications.

No patient had an increase in CPK-MB above normal limits. Postoperative LV ejection fraction was either unchanged (n = 3) or improved (n = 2, mean increase in LVEF = 5%). All patients were discharged on postoperative day 4 except one patient who remained in hospital for 72 days.

## Change in clinical status

All patients had a decrease in anginal frequency and severity. There was no change in the anginal pattern in any patient up to 10 days after gene transfer. All patients began to experience a reduction in angina between 10 and 30 days after gene transfer. Of 11 patients followed for more than 90 days, six (55%) were free of angina. The mean number of anginal episodes per week decreased from 50.1 ± 4.7 at baseline to 3.0 ± 1.9 at 90 days' follow-up (p < 0.0001). Use of sublingual nitroglycerine also decreased from 60.7 ± 5.9 tablets per week before treatment to 2.5 ± 2.0 per week after 90 days (p < 0.0001).

### Examples of patients enrolled

Patient 1 was a 67-year old man who was restricted to a wheelchair owing to a prior cerebrovascular accident. He had daily angina induced by mild activity such as movement in bed or transferring from bed to wheelchair, requiring an average of 8 NTG/day. All native vessels and 3/4 bypass grafts were occluded. Several institutions had advised the patient that the small caliber of his remaining native vessels precluded repeat CABG. His postoperative course after gene therapy was unremarkable. Beginning on postoperative day 21, the patient began to notice a decrease in the frequency and severity of his angina. By day 60 follow-up the patient no longer experienced anginal discomfort and no longer required NTG. He was able to engage in activities such as swimming, which were previously not possible due to anginal pain.

Patient 2, a 69-year-old man, had daily angina precipitated by mild activity such as walking about 10 yards, and had for several months been using 12 NTG/day. A vein graft to the left obtuse marginal (LOM) was occluded, and a diffusely diseased vein graft to a diagonal branch of the left anterior descending (LAD) coronary artery was not amenable to percutaneous revascularization. Additional surgery was not feasible because of poor target vessels. The patient's operative and perioperative courses were uncomplicated. Symptoms remained unchanged for around 3 weeks. The patient then began to notice a decrease in NTG consumption accompanied by the ability to increase his level of activity. By postoperative day 60 the patient was able to exercise on an exercise bicycle at his local gymnasium for up to 30 min. The patient's NTG requirement decreased to a maximum of 2 per day for occasional episodes of mild angina.

Patient 3, a 53-year-old man, had daily angina induced by walking for up to 50 yards, and used 6 NTG/day. All native vessels were occluded; grafts to the

LAD and right coronary artery (RCA) were patent, while an LOM graft was occluded. Percutaneous revascularization was not possible and a third bypass operation for single vessel bypass to a small-caliber target vessel was not feasible. Gene transfer and the perioperative course were unremarkable. The patients had no change in anginal symptoms until postoperative week 2, when he noticed an increase in the level of activity required to induce angina. At that time he was able to perform activities such as planting his garden that he had not previously engaged in for several months, and NTG use decreased to 5 per week. By 60 days after gene transfer he was able to walk up to half a mile without experiencing angina.

Patient 4, a 71-year-old man, complained of daily angina precipitated by minimal activity, including walking for less than 100 yards. All native vessels as well as grafts to the RCA and LOM were occluded. Percutaneous revascularization was not possible and repeat surgery was not feasible because of small-caliber target vessels. Gene therapy and postoperative recovery were uncomplicated. Beginning on day 10 after gene transfer, the patient noted increased exercise capacity accompanied by decreased NTG use. By follow-up day 30, the patient required no NTG and had returned to his 5 h per day job doing maintenance for his church. Between days 30 and 60, the patient developed fluid retention with dyspnea, associated with inadvertent discontinuation of his daily diuretic (furosemide 80 mg). After resumption of his diuretic, his symptoms resolved and he returned to his previous activity level without anginal symptoms, dyspnea, or NTG use.

Patient 5, a 59-year-old man with daily angina precipitated by activity such as walking 10–20 yards, also required continuous oxygen because of severe chronic obstructive pulmonary disease. He had been in hospital previously for several months because of intractable angina requiring intravenous NTG. All native vessels as well as vein grafts to RCA and diagonal branch of the LAD were occluded. Percutaneous revascularization was not possible, and a third bypass operation was not feasible due to poor distal vessels. Gene therapy and postoperative course were uncomplicated. By follow-up day 30 the patient noted that he was experiencing no angina and was able to walk distances of up to 500 yards. Additionally, he found that his use of supplemental oxygen had decreased. At 60 days' follow-up he reported a total of two anginal episodes in the previous month, each of which resolved with a single NTG tablet.

## SPECT sestamibi perfusion imaging

Perfusion imaging revealed significant improvement in myocardial perfusion on both stress and rest images. The perfusion/ischemia score during stress decreased from $21 \pm 1.8$ to $16.8 \pm 1.6$ ($p = 0.014$) while the ischemia score at rest decreased from $16.3 \pm 1.4$ to $12.4 \pm 1.4$ ($p = 0.027$).

## Coronary angiography

Selective coronary angiography was done before and 59.8 ± 1.5 days after gene transfer. Angiographic evidence for improved collateral flow into ischemia areas of the myocardium was observed in all patients. Five patients improved in one territory by 1–2 Rentrop grades, while seven patients improved in two territories by 1–3 Rentrop grades.

# Future directions

## Catheter-based myocardial gene transfer using non–fluoroscopic electromechanical LV mapping

While intravascular, pericardial, and intramuscular gene transfer have all been done by use of minimally invasive delivery techniques, intramyocardial gene transfer has to date required an operative thoractomy. Such an approach clearly implies additional morbidity, and limits the feasibility of repeat administrations. Successful execution of percutaneous, catheter-based myocardial gene transfer has not been previously reported.

Accordingly, we sought to investigate the safety and feasibility of a new delivery catheter for percutaneous myocardial gene transfer. To determine if the delivery catheter could be used in a site-specific manner, myocardial gene transfer was integrated with a previously described catheter mapping technology.[40] The results of this preliminary study indeed establish that percutaneous myocardial gene transfer can be successfully achieved in normal and ischemic myocardium in a relatively site-specific fashion, without significant morbidity or mortality. These findings thus establish the potential to replace current operative approaches with a minimally invasive technique for applications of cardiovascular gene therapy designed to target myocardial function.

## Methods

*Electromechanical LV mapping*
The NOGA system (Biosense, Johnson and Johnson) is designed to acquire, analyze, and display electroanatomical maps of the human heart. The maps are constructed by combining and integrating information from intracardiac electrograms acquired at multiple endocardial locations. Catheters designed for use with the NOGA system are equipped with an electromagnetic sensor, which provides real-time location of the catheter. As the catheter is moved along the endocardium, local endocardial electrograms, together with the catheter tip location, are reported simultaneously. The system then uses this information to

**141**

construct a three-dimensional (3D) electroanatomical map, which is a geometrical representation of the left ventricle (LV).

The NOGA system is designed to analyze global and local parameters that characterize mechanical, dynamic, and electrical LV function. Local functional analysis is based on local shortening as an index of local mechanical function, while measurement of local intracardiac signals determines viability based upon preserved electrical function. The combination of these data permits assessment of electromechanical coupling.

### NOGA components

The mapping and navigation system comprises a locator pad, a reference catheter, a mapping catheter, and a processing unit with a graphics computer (Silicon Graphics). A similar system, CARTO (Biosense), has been described previously in detail.[40,41]

The locator pad consists of a triangular arrangement of three magnetic coils, which together generate an ultralow intensity magnetic field (0.02G to 0.5G). The pad attaches to the undersurface of the catheterization table. The reference catheter (Cordis-Webster) is taped directly to the skin overlying the anterior or posterior chest wall within the frame of reference created by the three coils of the locator pad. It is used to detect small changes in intracardiac position due to respiration or movement of the subject. These small changes are analyzed by the computer to correct spatial information generated by the mapping catheter.

The mapping catheter (Cordis-Webster) is an 8F fused-tip catheter with a miniature passive magnetic field sensor embedded within its distal tip. Based on the strength of the magnetic field emitted from the locator pad coils, this sensor maps the distance from each coil; these distances determine the radii of theoretical spheres around each coil. The intersection of these three spheres determines the location and orientation of the sensor in 6 degrees of freedom (x, y, z, roll, pitch, and yaw), which thus indicates the position and rotation of the distal catheter segment. The accuracy of the sensor position in this low magnetic field is 0.8 mm and 5 degrees.[40,41] Unipolar or bipolar signals (timing related to a reference signal) are also obtained from the distal tip of the catheter, which allows generation of activation times in relation to the position of the catheter in the heart.

### Mapping procedure

The mapping procedure has been previously described in detail.[40,41] Briefly, the reference catheter was placed within the field of reference. The mapping catheter was introduced via a femoral arteriotomy and advanced to the LV. Three points (high septum, high lateral wall, apex) were obtained with fluoroscopic guidance to generate the initial 3D image of the LV. The location of the mapping catheter was gated to a reliable point in the cardiac cycle (recorded relative to the location of the fixed reference catheter at that time) and its location was continuously shown on the screen of the mapping computer. An icon of the mapping catheter was superimposed on the 3D map, thus enabling catheter manipulation in relation to the 3D map.

At each site, three parameters are calculated to determine the stability of endocardial contact with the catheter tip: location, cycle length (CL), and local activation time (LAT). Location is a measure of how stable the tip location is between beats. CL indicates the difference between the current CL and the median CL of the last 100 acquired points. LAT is calculated as the interval between a reliable point on the body-surface ECG and the steepest negative intrinsic deflection from the mapping-catheter unipolar recording, as determined from the intracardiac electrogram. This electrophysiological information is color-coded (red being the shortest LAT, purple being the longest) and superimposed on the 3D chamber geometry. The reconstruction is updated in real time with the acquisition of each new site. Validation of intracardiac signal recording and location accuracy, both in vitro and in vivo, have been previously established.[40,41]

*Injection catheter*
The injection catheter (Cordis-Webster) is a modified mapping catheter, the distal tip of which incorporates a 27G needle, which can be protruded by 3–5 mm. Map sites were acquired as described above, and superimposed upon the previously acquired 3D electroanatomical map. Once a stable point was attained, the needle was extended into the myocardium by 4–5 mm and the intracardiac electrogram monitored for myocardial injury and arrhythmias. After completion of the injection, the needle was retracted and the catheter moved to another endocardial site within the same target region.

In the current study, injection solutions were delivered according to one of three protocols as outlined below. Each injection consisted of 1 ml of solution (total volume = 6 per animal) delivered from a 1 ml syringe.

*Animal studies*
A total of 20 pigs weighing 30–50 kg were studied under protocols approved by the Animal Care and Use Committee of the St Elizabeth's Medical Center, in accordance with the Guide for the Care and Use of Laboratory Animals (Department of Health and Human Services, publication No. [NIH] 86–23 revised 1985).

NOGA mapping was done as previously described. An activation map was reconstructed from multiple LV endocardial sites. The injection catheter was then advanced to the LV, and injections were made according to three separate protocols. After six injections, the arteriotomy was closed and the pig was allowed to recover (except in protocol 1, in which the animals were immediately sacrificed).

**143**

## Results

*Mapping procedure*

During the mapping procedure, heart rate (pre-mapping $= 118 \pm 8$/min *vs* post-mapping $= 120 \pm 10$/min), systolic blood pressure ($92 \pm 3$ *vs* $87 \pm 4$ mmHg) and $O_2$ saturation ($98 \pm 0.5$ *vs* $99 \pm 0.4\%$) remained stable. Mapping was associated with transient ventricular ectopic activity but no sustained ventricular arrhythmias. No other complications were associated with the mapping procedure.

Activation (electroanatomical) maps of the LV during sinus rhythm were created in all pigs. All maps were completed in less than 20 min. The mean number of points acquired per map was $93 \pm 6$ (45–127). The site of earliest activation was in each case at the superior part of the septum (red/orange); the latest site of activation was on the left lateral wall close to the mitral valve apparatus (purple). Before injection, electromechanical interrogation was done, which consisted of maximum voltage (electrical activity) and linear log shortening (mechanical function) maps. Electrically viable tissue produced maximum unipolar voltage of more than 10 mV, and mechanically functional myocardium produced linear log shortening of more than 5%. In all non-ischemic pigs, both mechanical function and electrical activity were within normal limits. In the two pigs with an ameroid constrictor, evidence of myocardial ischemia was detected in the lateral wall by electromechanical uncoupling (high electrical voltage but low linear log shortening).

*Percutaneous LV gene transfer*

A total of 120 catheter-based injections were done in 20 pigs (six injections per animal). Percutaneous catheter-based myocardial injections caused no significant changes in heart rate (pre-injection $= 120 \pm 10$/min *vs* post-injection $= 128 \pm 11$/min), systolic blood pressure ($87 \pm 3$ *vs* $89 \pm 4$ mmHg), or $O_2$ saturation ($99 \pm 0.4$ *vs* $98 \pm 0.7\%$). Transient unifocal ventricular ectopic activity was observed at the time the needle was advanced into the myocardium. In all pigs, sporadic premature ventricular contractions occurred during injection. No episodes of sustained ventricular or atrial arrhythmias occurred. No injury pattern was observed during the injections as recorded by endocardial electrography. Likewise, the surface ECG showed no evidence of myocardial infarction in any pig. All pigs survived until sacrifice, and no complications, including pericardial effusion and cardiac tamponade, were observed in any animals.

*Protocol 1.* Six discrete sites of methylene blue staining, located in three LV myocardial areas (anteroapical, two; septum, two; posterolateral wall, two) were identified at necropsy in each heart. These sites corresponded to the injection sites indicated prospectively in vivo on the endocardial map. Myocardial staining was 5.2 $\pm$ 1.7 mm in depth and 6.4 $\pm$ 0.7 mm in width. No epicardial staining was demonstrated. In addition, X-gal staining produced no evidence of nuclear specific $\beta$-galactosidase activity in the myocardium at these sites; these two hearts thus constituted negative controls (since no gene transfer was done in either case) for protocol 2, below.

*Protocol 2.* The injection catheter was used to deliver pCMV-nls*LacZ* (50 µg/ml) to a single LV myocardial region in six pigs (apex, two; septum, two; posterolateral wall, one; anterior wall, one). In each of the six pigs, peak $\beta$-galactosidase activity after 5 days (RLU, mean = 135 333 $\pm$ 28 239 [31 508 $-$ 192 748]) was recorded in the target area of myocardial injection. Adjacent myocardial areas showed low level activity, and areas remote from the injection sites had negligible activity. Thus, percutaneous LV myocardial gene transfer was directed in a relatively localized fashion to those sites indicated by pre-injection electroanatomical mapping.

*Protocol 3.* Percutaneous gene transfer of pCMV-nls*LacZ* (50 µg/ml) was also done in two pigs in which an ameroid constrictor had applied to the left circumflex coronary artery. Myocardial ischemia, as evidenced by uncoupling of the mechanical and electrical parameters on endocardial mapping, was demonstrated in the lateral wall of both pigs. In each of the two pigs, peak $\beta$-galactosidase activity after 5 days (214 851 and 23 140 RLU) was documented in the target area of myocardial injection. As in the non-ischemic hearts, $\beta$-galactosidase activity was markedly diminished in tissue sections retrieved from adjacent myocardium and was negligible at remote sites.

## Pathology examination

*Gross examination.* In no case did gross examination disclose evidence of pericardial fluid or blood, epicardial hemorrhage or subendocardial hemorrhage. There was no evidence of perforation or tissue excavation. No vegetations were seen, nor were intracavitary thrombi observed.

*Microscopic examination.* Light microscopic examination was done on a total of 1500 slides (m = 75/heart) cut from the anterior, posterior, septal, and free walls of "breadloaf" slices of the left ventricle, and subsequently stained with hematoxylin and eosin. In non-ischemic hearts, rare foci of mononuclear cells were occasionally observed at sites of gene injection, but were also seen, though less often, in non-injected sites. In hearts in which myocardial ischemia was induced by placement of an ameroid constrictor around the left circumflex coronary artery, foci of fibrosis and mononuclear cell infiltrates were routinely observed at those sites subserved by the constricted artery. In the sites remote from the site of intended ischemia, rare foci of inflammatory cells were again observed. Occasional sites of limited interstitial erythrocyte extravasation were also observed.

**145**

# Discussion

These experiments suggest that myocardial gene transfer is indeed feasible and is safe in normal and ischemic myocardium of pigs. Injection of methylene blue was successfully achieved at six of six sites in two pigs. The extent of transmural distribution was limited to the LV wall, as shown by the absence of epicardial staining. Maximum gene expression was localized to the injection site in all pigs, ischemic as well as normal, injected with pCMV-nls*LacZ*. Myocardium adjacent to the target sites of injection showed low-level β-galactosidase activity, indicating limited distribution after gene transfer. All remote non-injected areas of myocardium were essentially devoid of β-galactosidase activity.

While the mapping capabilities of the NOGA system used in this study were useful to show that gene expression could be directed to specific LV sites, these findings do not establish that LV endocardial mapping is required for percutaneous myocardial gene transfer. Electroanatomical mapping may be advantageous since avoiding gene transfer to sites of myocardial scar can be avoided, and the tip of the injection catheter can be accurately relocated to areas of myocardial ischemia (or hibernating myocardium) where gene transfer may be potentially optimized.[32] Theoretically, adjunctive mapping could be employed in a serial fashion to gauge the success of certain gene therapy strategies (eg, therapeutic angiogenesis). These potential advantages, however, will require further documentation and assessment of physiological improvement after delivery of a non-reporter gene to establish the value of adjunctive mapping.

Based on these data, a phase I trial of percutaneous intramyocardial VEGF gene therapy is scheduled to begin in the spring of 1999.

# References

1. Folkman J. Tumor angiogenesis: therapeutic implications *N Engl J Med* 1971; **285:** 1182–6.

2. Shing Y, Folkman J, Sullivan J et al. Heparin-affinity purification of a tumor-derived capillary endothelial cell growth factor. *Science* 1984; **223:** 1296–9.

3. White FC, Carroll SM, Magnet A, Bloor CM. Coronary collateral development in swine after coronary artery occlusion. *Circ Res* 1992; **71:** 1490–500.

4. Baffour R, Berman J, Garb JL et al. Enhanced angiogenesis and growths of collaterals by in vivo administration of recombinant basic fibroblast growth factor in a rabbit model of acute lower limb ischemia: dose-response effect of basic fibroblast growth factor. *J Vasc Surg* 1992; **16:** 181–91.

5. Pu LQ, Sniderman AD, Brassard R et al. Enhanced revascularization of the ischemic limb by means of angiogenic therapy. *Circulation* 1993; **88:** 208–15.

6.    Yanagisawa-Miwa A, Uchida Y, Nakamura F et al. Salvage of infarcted myocardium by angiogenic action of basic fibroblast growth factor. *Science* 1992; **257:** 1401–3.

7.    Ferrara N, Henzel WJ. Pituitary follicular cells secrete a novel heparin-binding growth factor specific for vascular endothelial cells. *Biochem Biophys Res Commun* 1989; **161:** 851–5.

8.    Keck PJ, Hausser SD, Krivi G et al. Vascular permeability factor, an endothelial cell mitogen related to PDGF. *Science* 1989; **246:** 1309–12.

9.    Connolly DR, Olander JV, Heuvelman D et al. Human vascular permeability factor: isolation from U937 cells. *J Biol Chem* 1989; **264:** 20017–24.

10.   Leung DW, Cachianes G, Kuang WJ et al. Vascular endothelial growth factor is a secreted angiogenic mitogen. *Science* 1989; **246:** 1306–9.

11.   de Vries C, Escobedo JA, Ueno H. The *fms*-like tyrosine kinase, a receptor for vascular endothelial growth factor. *Science* 1992; **255:** 989–91.

12.   Millauer B, Wizigmann-Voos S, Schnurch H et al. High affinity VEGF binding and developmental expression suggest *Flk*-1 as a major regulator of vasculogenesis and angiogenesis. *Cell* 1993; **72:** 835–46.

13.   Terman BI. Dougher-Vermazen M, Carrion ME et al. Identification of the KDR tyrosine kinase as a receptor for vascular endothelial cell growth factor. *Biochem Biophys Res Commun* 1992; **187:** 1579–86.

14.   Klagsbrun M, D'Amore PA. Regulators of angiogenesis. *Annu Rev Physiol* 1991; **53:** 217–39.

15.   Gospodarowicz D, Massoglia S, Cheng J, Fujii DK. Effect of fibroblast growth factor and lypoproteins on the proliferation of endothelial cells derived from bovine adrenal cortex, brain cortex, and corpus luteum capillaries. *J Cell Physiol* 1986; **127:** 121–36.

16.   Conn G, Soderman D, Schaeffer M-T et al. Purification of glycoprotein vascular endothelial cell mitogen from a rat glioma cell line. *Proc Natl Acad Sci USA* 1990; **87:** 1323–7.

17.   Shen H, Clauss M, Ryan J et al. Characterization of vascular permeability factor/vascular endothelial growth factor receptors on mononuclear phagocytes. *Blood* 1993; **81:** 2767–73.

18.   Clauss M, Gerlach M, Gerlach H et al. Vascular permeability factor: a tumor-derived polypeptide that induces endothelial cell and monocyte procoagulant activity, and promotes monocyte migration. *J Exp Med* 1990; **172:** 1535–45.

19.   Levy AP, Tamargo R, Brem H, Nathans D. An endothelial cell growth factor from the mouse neuroblastoma cell line NB41. *Growth Factors* 1989; **2:** 9–19.

20.   Connolly DT, Hewelman DM, Nelson R et al. Tumor vascular permeability factor stimulates endothelial cell growth and angiogenesis. *J Clin Invest* 1989; **84:** 1470–8.

**147**

21. Takeshita S, Zheng LP, Asahara T et al. Therapeutic angiogenesis: a single intra-arterial bolus of vascular endothelial growth factor augments collateral vessel formation in a rabbit ischemic hindlimb. *Circulation* 1993; **88:** I–370 (abstr).

22. Takeshita S, Pu L-Q, Zheng L et al. Vascular endothelial growth factor induces dose-dependent revascularization in a rabbit model of persistent limb ischemia. *Circulation* 1994; **90:** II-228–II-234.

23. Isner JM, Kaufman J, Rosenfield K et al. Combined physiologic and anatomic assessment of percutaneous revascularization using a Doppler guidewire and ultrasound catheter. *Am J Cardiol* 1993; **71:** 70D–86D.

24. Bauters C, Asahara T, Zheng LP et al. Physiologic assessment of augmented vascularity induced by VEGF in ischemic rabbit hindlimb. *Am J Physiol* 1994; **267:** H1263–71.

25. Losordo DW, Pickering JG, Takeshita S et al. Use of the rabbit ear artery to serially assess foreign protein secretion after site specific arterial gene transfer in vivo: evidence that anatomic identification of successful gene transfer may underestimate the potential magnitude of transgene expression. *Circulation* 1994; **89:** 785–92.

26. Riessen R, Rahimizadeh H, Blessing E et al. Arterial gene transfer using pure DNA applied directly to a hydrogel-coated angioplasty balloon. *Hum Gene Ther* 1993; **4:** 749–58.

27. Isner JM, Pieczek A, Schainfeld R et al. Clinical evidence of angiogenesis following arterial gene transfer of phVEGF$_{165}$. *Lancet* 1996; **348:** 370–4.

28. Nabel EG, Plautz G, Nabel GJ. Transduction of a foreign histocompatibility gene into the arterial wall induces vasculitis. *Proc Natl Acad Sci USA* 1992; **89:** 5157–61.

29. Nabel EG, Yang Z, Liptay S et al. Recombinant platelet-derived growth factor B gene expression in porcine arteries induces intimal hyperplasia in vivo. *J Clin Invest* 1993; **91:** 1822–9.

30. Nabel EG, Yang ZY, Plautz G et al. Recombinant fibroblast growth factor-1 promotes intimal hyperplasia and angiogenesis in arteries *in vivo*. *Nature* 1993; **362:** 844–6.

31. Takeshita S, Losordo DW, Kearney M, Isner JM. Time course of recombinant protein secretion following liposome-mediated gene transfer in a rabbit arterial organ culture model. *Lab Invest* 1994; **71:** 387–91.

32. Tsurumi Y, Takeshita S, Chen D et al. Direct intramuscular gene transfer of naked DNA encoding vascular endothelial growth factor augments collateral development and tissue perfusion. *Circulation* 1996; **94:** 3281–90.

33. Takeshita S, Isshiki T, Sato T. Increased expression of direct gene transfer into skeletal muscles observed after acute ischemic injury in rats. *Lab Invest* 1996; **74:** 1061–5.

**148**

34. Gal D, Weir L, Leclerc G et al. Direct myocardial transfection in two animal models: evaluation of parameters affecting gene expression and percutaneous gene delivery. *Lab Invest* 1993; **68:** 18–25.

35. Oswald H, Heinemann F, Nikol S et al. Removal of an inhibitor of marker enzyme activity in artery extracts by chelating agents. *Biotechniques* 1997; **22:** 78–81.

36. Tsurumi Y, Murohara T, Krasinski K et al. Reciprocal relationship between VEGF and NO in the regulation of endothelial integrity. *Nature Med* 1997; **3:** 879–86.

37. Tischer E, Mitchell R, Hartmann T et al. The human gene for vascular endothelial growth factor: multiple protein forms are encoded through alternative exon splicing. *J Biol Chem* 1991; **266:** 11947–54.

38. Baumgartner I, Pieczek A, Manor O et al. Constitutive expression of phVEGF$_{165}$ following intramuscular gene transfer promotes collateral vessel development in patients with critical limb ischemia. *Circulation* 1998; **97:** 1114–23.

39. Rentrop KP, Cohen M, Blanke H, Phillips RA. Changes in coronary collateral filling immediately after controlled coronary artery occlusion by an angioplasty balloon in human subjects. *J Am Coll Cardiol* 1985; **5:** 587–92.

40. Gepstein L, Hayman G, Ben-Haim SA. A novel method for nonfluoroscopic catheter-based electroanatomical mapping of the heart: in vitro and in vivo accuracy results. *Circulation* 1997; **95:** 1611–22.

41. Ben-Haim SA, Osadchy, Schuster I et al. Nonfluoroscopic, in vivo navigation and mapping technology. *Nature Med* 1996; **2:** 1393–5.

**149**

# 12. Biological Revascularization Using Adenovirus Coding for Vascular Endothelial Growth Factor 121

Leonard Y Lee, Kenneth T Lee, Ronald G Crystal and Todd K Rosengart

## Introduction

Atherosclerosis and ischemic heart disease, the leading causes of death in developed countries, have long been treated by such interventions as percutaneous transluminal coronary angioplasty (PTCA) and coronary artery bypass grafting (CABG).[1] Recently, therapeutic angiogenesis has emerged as a potential therapy for a growing number of patients who are not candidates for conventional therapies secondary to anatomical constraints imposed by the severity or extent of their coronary artery disease (CAD). "Therapeutic angiogenesis" describes the process of new blood vessel formation induced by specific mediator proteins referred to as "angiogens". Under normal circumstances, ischemia results in the upregulation of these growth factors, although this response is often not robust enough to mediate therapeutic angiogenesis.[2] This presents the optimal setting for "biological revascularization", in which an angiogen is administered therapeutically to stimulate new vascularization and enhance perfusion of ischemic tissues.[3]

A large body of work pertaining to therapeutic angiogenesis now exists, including assessments of therapeutic efficacy of the many known candidate angiogenic growth factors in a large number of animal models, and assessments of several techniques for delivering these growth factors to target tissues. Many extensive reviews of this literature have now been published, which provide comprehensive summaries of the field. For the purposes of this report, we have focused on a series of decision points that were reached and crossed, based upon the available data in the literature or our own studies, that led us to use direct myocardial injection of an adenovirus coding for the 121 amino acid isoform of vascular endothelial growth factor (Ad$_{GV}$VEGF121.10) to induce myocardial angiogenesis. These decision points included choices of the optimal growth factor, delivery vehicle (protein *vs* gene therapy, and type of vector to be used), delivery strategy (systemic *vs* local), and, finally, delivery technique (intracoronary *vs* intramyocardial). Although it is not known whether any of these options give therapeutic advantages, we believe that the rationale for these decisions is informative.

## Vascular endothelial growth factor

Vascular endothelial growth factor (VEGF; also referred to as VEGF-A or VEGA-1) is a homodimeric 34 to 46 kDa glycoprotein that is a critical contributor to vascular development in the embryo and a potent stimulator of angiogenesis in the post-natal state.[4] A family of VEGF proteins, including VEGF-B, C, D, E, and F, has been elucidated, which possesses similar sequence homology.

The receptors of VEGF, KDR/flk-1 and flt-1, are tyrosine kinase receptors with seven extracellular immunoglobulin-like domains.[5,6] These receptors are expressed almost exclusively on endothelial cells, which are capable of binding to all isoforms of VEGF (Table 12.1). Critical binding sites for VEGF are the amino acids Asp (63), Glu (64), and Glu (67) on KDR/flk-1, and the residues Arg (82), Lys (84) and His (86) on flt-1 localized to the 2nd and 3rd immunoglobulin chain of respective receptors.[5,6] Because of the localization of the VEGF receptors

**Table 12.1 Vascular endothelial growth factor (VEGF) isoforms and relative affinity to VEGF tyrosine kinase receptors**

|  | Receptors Flt-1 | KDR/Flk-1 | Flt-4 |
|---|---|---|---|
| VEGF121 | +++ | 0 | 0 |
| VEGF165 | ++ | ++ | ND |
| VEGF189 | ND | ND | ND |
| VEGF206 | ND | ND | ND |
| VEGF-B | ++ | + | ND |
| VEGF-C | 0 | + | +++ |
| VEGF-D | 0 | ++ | ++ |
| VEGF-E | 0 | ++ | ND |
| VEGF-F | ND | ND | ND |

+ = minimal affinity, ++ = strong affinity, +++ = very strong affinity, ND = not determined.

primarily to the endothelial cell, VEGF is the most selective of the angiogenic growth factors. By contrast, other growth factors, such as the fibroblast growth factors, are mitogenic for a wide variety of other cell types including fibroblasts, and thus pose a theoretical risk for inducing unwanted fibrosis or myointimal hyperplasia. This consideration represents the basis of our selection of VEGF as our therapeutic angiogen.

The human VEGF gene normally expresses four different isoforms of VEGF, secondary to post-transcriptional mRNA splicing, producing VEGF proteins of 121, 165, 189, and 206 amino acid residues.[4] All isoforms, with the exception of VEGF121, bind to heparan proteoglycans in the extracellular matrix and heparin. As a result, VEGF121 theoretically has the greatest ability to diffuse through tissues from the original site of protein elaboration. It was ultimately the isoform selected for our advanced preclinical studies as well as our clinical trial.

## Gene therapy versus protein therapy

Several angiogen delivery strategies have been developed to maximize efficacy of this therapy while minimizing toxic effects. These delivery techniques can be subclassified into two basic delivery strategies; protein therapy and gene therapy. Both therapies have been shown to induce angiogenesis in animal models, and have been advanced to clinical trials.

Protein therapy consists of the delivery of pharmacological dosages of angiogenic proteins either systemically, or targeted to tissues locally, to induce angiogenesis. Systemic protein-delivery strategies may be limited in terms of efficacy, however, by the short half life of angiogenic growth factors, and by potential toxic side-effects such as hypotension associated with the systemic administration of these growth factors, and the possibilities of promiscuous angiogenesis in sites remote from the targeted tissue, such as occult tumors or the retina.[7] To increase the localized efficacy of protein-based delivery strategies, relatively cumbersome techniques such as sustained-release polymers (eg, heparin-alginate beads) and catheter/reservoir systems have been devised.[8–10]

With the increasing success of vector development, permitting successful gene transfer in a number of animal models, gene therapy has emerged as a new strategy for delivery of angiogens to targeted tissues. Gene therapy is usually provided by the single administration of a vector that contains an expression cassette consisting of a promoter modulating expression of the gene, the cDNA of interest, and appropriate stop signals to end translation.[11,12] The vector transfers the gene of interest, or transgene, to targeted cells, which then produce the corresponding protein product. The various vector systems available – either a simple DNA sequence (plasmid) or a replication deficient virus (adenovirus, adeno-associated virus, retrovirus) – transfer expression cassettes through mechanisms that differ in terms of duration and susceptibility of target cell types of transgene expression and thus have distinct advantages and disadvantages depending upon the desired expression profile. All gene-therapy-based strategies take advantage, however, of the sustained expression of cellular-derived growth factor that is produced upon transfection of targeted cells by an appropriate vector. Furthermore, it has been shown in several models that by injecting an appropriate vector directly into targeted tissues, the distribution of the expressed transgene can be restricted to the area of vector administration. Thus, gene therapy, which we chose to use as a delivery strategy, is a means of delivering sustained, localized expression of a selected transgene. Currently, only plasmids and adenoviruses have been used in clinical myocardial angiogenesis trials.

## Adenovirus vectors

Adenoviruses (Ad) are DNA viruses comprised of a 36 kb linear, double stranded DNA genome, and core proteins surrounded by capsid proteins. There are 49 human Ad serotypes identified, categorized into six subgroups based on DNA homology.[13] The subgroup C viruses, serotypes 2 and 5, are the best characterized and are the basis for gene transfer vectors in current use for preclinical and clinical studies of Ad-mediated gene transfer. By rendering the virus replication deficient, by deleting the E1 region in the viral genome and inserting the exogenous gene of interest with an appropriate promoter, the Ad vector is then capable of transferring up to 7 kb of foreign DNA into targeted cells or tissues.[14]

---

***Figure 12.1:*** *Expression of VEGF in the retroperitoneal fat pad of Sprague-Dawley rats. Dose was $10^9$ pfu; the arrow indicates the time of vector administration; the first timepoint represents naive tissue, and the second timepoint tissue immediately after vector administration. (a) Quantification of VEGF expression in retroperitoneal adipose tissue by enzyme-linked immunoassay over time following local administration of the AdCMV.VEGF vector. Data are shown for the AdCMV.VEGF vector and AdCMV.Null vector.*
*(b) Quantification of neovascularization of adipose tissue over time after administration of AdCMV.VEGF to adipose tissue. Number of blood vessels observed in vivo at the macroscopic level (30✕) is shown over time for AdCMV.VEGF, AdCMV.Null control, sham control, and untreated adipose tissue after administration of AdCMV.VEGF to contralateral retroperitoneal adipose tissue.*
*(c) Quantification of capillary number of adipose tissue over time after administration of AdCMV.VEGF. Capillary numbers per $mm^2$ are shown over time for AdCMV.VEGF, AdCMV.Null vectors. (Reproduced with permission from Magovern et al[17].)*

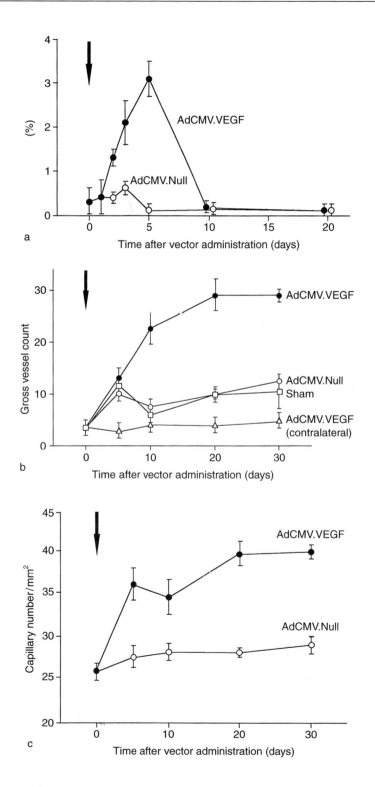

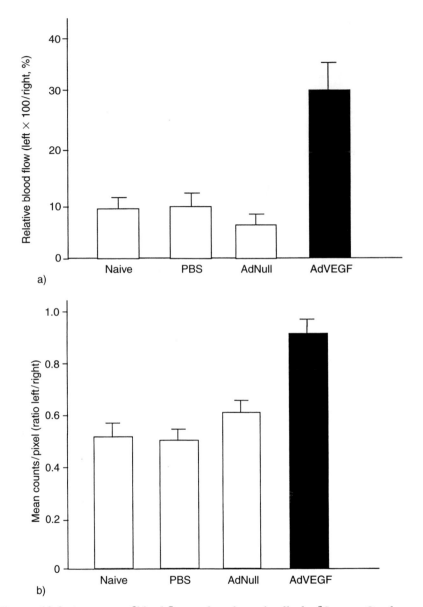

**Figure 12.2:** *Assessment of blood flow in the ischemic hindlimb of Sprague-Dawley rats. (a) Relative blood flow assessed with color microspheres in hindlimbs. After ligation of the femoral artery, color microspheres were injected into the infrarenal aorta. Relative blood flow is expressed as microspheres per g tissue in the ligated hindlimb (left) versus microspheres per g tissue in the contralateral (right) hindlimb. (b) Relative blood flow assessed by $^{99m}Tc$-labeled sestamibi imaging in hindlimbs immediately after ligation of left femoral artery. Relative blood flow is quantified as the ratio of left versus right geometric mean counts per pixel of dorsal and ventral*

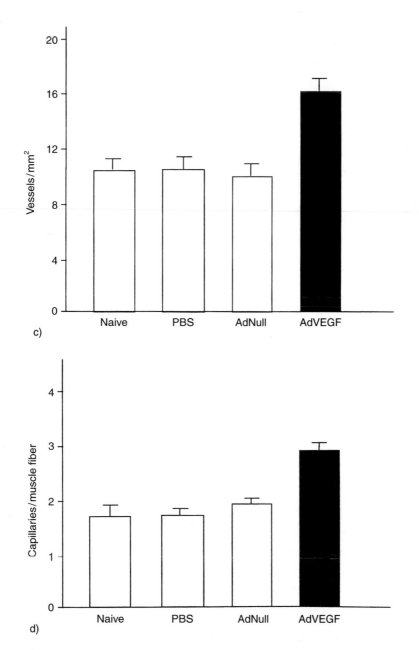

c)

d)

*views of the calf of the ligated hindlimb (left) to the same area of the contralateral hindlimb (right).*

*(c) Histological quantification of small-vessel (less than 80 μm diameter) count expressed as mean number of vessels per mm².*

*(d) Histological quantification of capillary number in skeletal muscle shown as capillaries per muscle fiber. (Reproduced with permission from Mack et al[18].)*

**157**

Due to host immune responses, the expression of Ad vectors is limited to a period of days to weeks.[15] For purposes of therapeutic angiogenesis, this feature of Ad vectors may be ideal in that it provides adequate duration of angiogen expression for angiogenesis to occur, but is limited to an extent that may prevent derangement of blood vessel growth.[16] In contrast to the use of an Ad vector, plasmids are not limited by issues of immunogenicity, but possess about $10^3$–$10^4$-fold lower transection efficiency. Based upon these considerations, we used an Ad vector as our gene-therapy delivery vehicle.

## Preclinical experiments

### Preliminary studies

First, we validated the efficacy of gene transfer by use of an Ad vector encoding the human form of VEGF165 (AdVEGF165) by direct injection of this vector into the retroperitoneal fat pad of Sprague-Dawley rats.[17] The retroperitoneal fat pad is an ideal bioassay to assess the efficacy of blood vessel growth secondary to its relatively avascular composition. These studies showed high levels of VEGF protein expression localized to the regional adipose tissues of AdVEGF treated animals compared with appropriate controls (Figure 12.1a). The lack of systemic "spillover" was shown by the absence of increases in VEGF amounts in the serum or in distant organs. Furthermore, the expression of AdVEGF165 was limited to 10 days after injection of the vector. Comparisons of adipose tissue injected with AdNull (control vector) and AdVEGF165 treated animals showed a time-dependent increase of over 100% in macroscopic vessel number, beginning at 10 days after vector administration and plateauing by 30 days after vector administration (Figure 12.1b). Histological examination of samples showed about a 40% increase in microscopic vessel numbers in the AdVEGF165 versus AdNull fat pads (Figure 12.1c).

Once the effectiveness of AdVEGF in inducing blood vessel growth was confirmed in non-ischemic tissues, the efficacy of the same vector to correct an ischemic state was assessed in a rat hindlimb model.[18] Increased blood flow was noted in the iliac artery ligated animals receiving AdVEGF165 compared with AdNull treated animals, as documented by microsphere injections (Figure 12.2a), and single photon emission computerized tomography-SPECT with [99m]technetium labeled sestamibi scans (Figure 12.2b). Angiographic and histological evidence of increased vascularity and capillary number in local adipose tissue and per muscle fiber was also noted in the AdVEGF treated groups (Figure 12.2c, d). In addition, treatment with AdVEGF protected against a rise in femoral vein lactate levels, an indicator of anaerobic respiration, 1 h after acute femoral artery ligation.

**158**

## Myocardial gene transfer

The feasibility of direct myocardial gene transfer was investigated in canine hearts, characterizing the spatial and temporal limits of the replication-deficient adenovirus with direct myocardial injections.[19] In these studies, two different Ad vectors were used: one containing the gene coding for chloramphenicol acetyl transferase (AdCAT), and a second containing the gene coding for human VEGF165 (AdVEGF165). Transgene expression in myocardium was found in a zone around the injection site about 10 mm in diameter, which was surrounded by a peripheral zone of decreased expression 11–15 mm from the original injection site. CAT activity persisted at levels significantly higher than baseline for about 14 days, with the central zone showing twice the gene expression of peripheral zones. CAT activity was assessed in distant organ systems and was less than 0.1% of the expression of the injected left ventricle. The AdVEGF165 vector produced VEGF expression that peaked at 2 days and persisted above baseline for some 14 days after vector delivery.

A critical decision point involved a comparison of direct intramyocardial administration of Ad vectors with intracoronary delivery of the same Ad vectors. For this comparison, a catheter-based intracoronary administration via femoral artery catheterization was done with a 7F 100 cm catheter, which was advanced under fluoroscopic guidance to the left coronary ostium and positioned in the proximal left anterior descending artery. AdCAT ($10^9$ pfu) in 1 ml phosphate buffered saline was injected over 10 s and flushed with 3 ml of 0.9% NaCl. The results showed minimal myocardial expression of AdCAT compared with those animals that received the Ad vector by direct myocardial injection (same total dose as 10 injections, same total volume, Figure 12.3). These preliminary studies culminated in the assessment of the efficacy and toxicity of a clinical grade Ad vector coding for VEGF to mediate therapeutic angiogenesis in a model of myocardial ischemia using direct myocardial injection.

## Therapeutic angiogenesis in the heart

For studies of efficacy and toxic effects, the clinical grade Ad vector coding for the VEGF121 isoform ($Ad_{GV}VEGF121.10$-GenVec, Rockville, MD) was used in a porcine model of chronic myocardial ischemia.[20] Ischemia in the circumflex distribution was established by placement of 2.5 mm internal diameter ameroid constrictor (Research Instruments & MFG, Corvaillis, OR) on the left circumflex coronary artery via left thoractomy. After 3 weeks (time sufficient to allow for induction of ischemia), the therapeutic vector $Ad_{GV}VEGF121.10$ was injected into the region of ischemia as 10 doses of $10^8$ pfu in 100 μl in each (total $10^9$ pfu/1000 μl) and compared with animals that received the AdNull control. No differences were notable at the time of vector administration, 3 weeks after

**159**

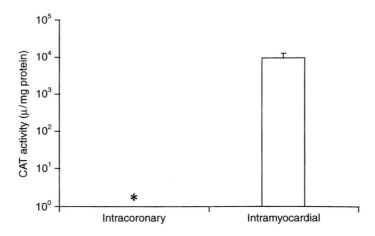

*Figure 12.3:* Comparison of intracoronary versus intramyocardial delivery of AdCAT in the canine myocardium. Myocardium was harvested 2 days after vector administration and the relative CAT activity was determined. Results are means ± SEM: the black bar represents intracoronary delivery and the open bar represents intramyocardial delivery. The asterisk represents a value below the threshold of detectability.

ameroid (Figure 12.4a). However, a significant reduction in the region of ischemia was shown 4 weeks after vector administration and 7 weeks after ameroid placement, by SPECT with [99m]technetium labeled sestamibi (Figure 12.4b). Furthermore, stress echocardiography showed improvement in segmental wall thickening in the ischemic region when compared with controls with near normalization of ventricular function in the treated group (Figure 12.4c). Near complete reconstitution of the left circumflex coronary artery distribution was achieved in treated animals via collateral vessel formation, as shown by ex-vivo angiography (Figure 12.4d).

In a concurrent series of experiments, the safety of Ad vector coding for VEGF was established in a similar porcine model.[21] High dose (10-fold greater than the dose used to show efficacy) vector administration into ischemic myocardium of pigs showed no deterioration of myocardial function or increase in pericardial effusions as assessed by echocardiography. In addition, histological examination of livers, hearts, and other distant organs demonstrated minimal inflammation and necrosis at this high dose of vector. Blood analyses showed no significant abnormalities, similar to the results seen with the therapeutic dose.

An additional study was done in C57/B16 mice to assess the effects of intravenous administration of the same vector.[21] Toxic effects, manifested by

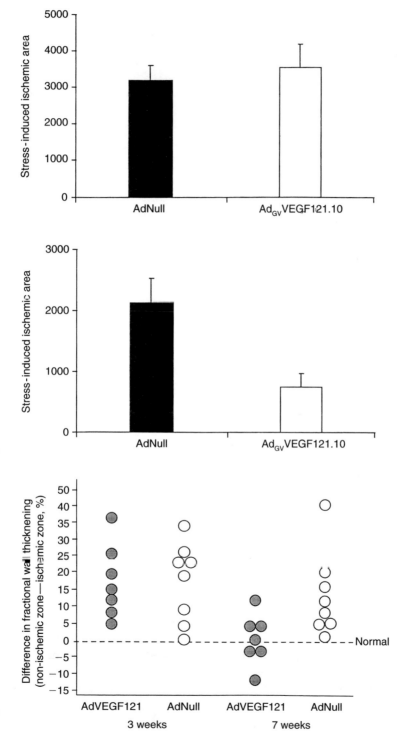

a

b

c

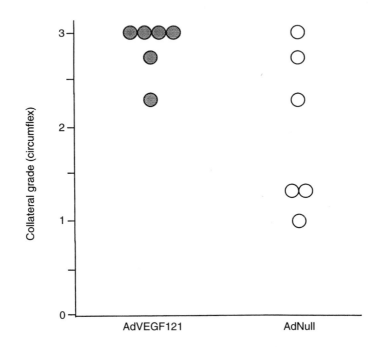

d

**Figure 12.4:** *Stress-induced ischemic area of myocardium of Yorkshire pigs.*
*(a) At vector administration, 3 weeks after ameroid.*
*(b) 4 weeks after vector administration, 7 weeks after ameroid. Ischemic area was determined by* $^{99m}Tc$*-sestamibi nuclear medicine scans at the time of vector administration and at the time of sacrifice, 7 weeks after ameroid. Results are means* $\pm$ *SEM: the black bar represents AdNull and the open bar represents* $Ad_{GV}VEGF121.10.$
*(c) Fractional wall thickening as assessed by echocardiography under stress conditions (rapid atrial pacing) calculated as mean systolic wall thickening/mean diastolic wall thickness.*
*(d) Rentrop scores as determined at the time of ex-vivo angiography where 0 = no filling of the circumflex coronary artery, 1 = filling of collateral branches without visualization of the epicardial segment; 2 and 3 = partial or complete filling of the epicardial segment of the circumflex coronary artery, respectively.*

increased mortality, hepatic inflammation and necrosis, and anemia were only evident in the highest dosage group ($10^{10}$ pfu, $10^3$-fold higher by weight than the efficacious dose in pigs). Combined with the lack of toxicity in pigs even at a dose 10-fold higher than the efficacious dose, these findings prompted a phase I clinical trial with the same clinical grade $Ad_{GV}VEGF121.10.$

**162**

# Clinical trials

With the evident safety and efficacy of Ad-mediated gene therapy in therapeutic angiogenesis in a porcine model of myocardial ischemia and a rat model of peripheral ischemia, a phase I study was begun (Rosengart et al[22]). This study consisted of two groups of patients, group A receiving $Ad_{GV}VEGF121.10$ as a dose escalation ($4 \times 10^8 - 4 \times 10^{10}$ pu) in $\frac{1}{2}$ log increments beginning with the lowest dose (n = 3/dose, total 15 patients) as an adjunct to conventional bypass surgery, and group B receiving $Ad_{GV}VEGF121.10$ ($4 \times 10^9$ pu) as sole therapy (n = 6). In general, the inclusion and exclusion criteria were similar for the two groups. The patients were men and women with an age range of 40 to 85 years who had reversible myocardial ischemia by dobutamine stress echocardiography, rest and stress $^{99m}Tc$-sestamibi nuclear medicine scans, and exercise tolerance tests.

As detailed in the study by Rosengart et al[22], there was no evidence of apparent systemic or cardiac-related adverse events related to vector administration. There was an improvement in angina class when comparing 30 days post vector with baseline values both in group A (assessed as a single cohort) and group B. Similarly, there were trends towards improvement in perfusion, as assessed by angiography, nuclear medicine studies, and exercise tolerance tests.

The results of this phase I clinical trial show that it is feasible and safe to use an Ad vector to deliver the coding sequence of the 121 amino acid form of VEGF to the myocardium of individuals with clinically significant coronary artery disease. Although the data from this phase I study are encouraging, larger phase II/III trials will be required to definitively assess the safety and efficacy of this therapy.

# Conclusions

Gene therapy and therapeutic angiogenesis hold promise for the treatment of patients with severe CAD not amenable to standard therapies such as CABG or PTCA. The experience thus far with direct myocardial injection of the $Ad_{GV}VEGF121.10$ vector is encouraging. With the advent of next-generation vectors, incorporating promoters such as cardiac specific or regulatable promoters, the clinician should someday be able to tailor the myocardial gene therapy for the treatment of disease-specific problems such as heart failure, or for the treatment of graft closure years after the initial surgical procedure.

# References

1.  Centers for Disease Control and Prevention. Trends in ischemic heart disease deaths – United States, 1990–1994. *JAMA* 1997; **277:** 1109.

2.  Banai S, Shweiki D, Pinson A et al. Upregulation of vascular endothelial growth factor expression induced by myocardial ischemia: implications for coronary angiogenesis. *Cardiovasc Res* 1994; **28:** 1176–9.

3.  Folkman J, Shing Y: Angiogenesis. *J Biol Chem* 1992; **267:** 10931–4.

4.  Ferrara N, Houck K, Jakeman L et al. The vascular endothelial growth factor family of polypeptides. *J Cell Biochem* 1991; **47:** 211–8.

5.  Shibuya M, Yamaguchi S, Yamane A et al. Nucleotide sequence and expression of a novel human receptor-type tyrosine kinase gene (flt) closely related to the fms family. *Oncogene* 1990; **5:** 519–24.

6.  Terman B, Dougher-Vermazen M, Carrion M et al. Identification of the KDR tyrosine kinase as a receptor for vascular endothelial growth factor. *Biochem Biophys Res Commun* 1992; **187:** 1579–86.

7.  Folkman J. Angiogenesis in cancer, vascular, rheumatoid and other diseases. *Nature Med* 1995; **1:** 27–31.

8.  Chleboun JO, Martins RN, Mitchell CA, Chrilla TV. Basic FGF enhances the development of the collateral circulation after acute arterial occlusion. *Biochem Biophys Res Commun* 1992; **185:** 510–6.

9.  Harada K, Friedman M, Lopez JJ et al. Vascular endothelial growth factor administration in chronic myocardial ischemia. *Am J Physiol* 1996; **270:** H1791–802.

10. Banai S, Jaklitsch MT, Casscells W et al. Effects of acidic fibroblast growth factor on normal and ischemic myocardium. *Circ Res* 1991; **69:** 76–85.

11. Takeshita S, Yukio T, Thierry C et al. Gene transfer of naked DNA encoding for three isoforms of vascular endothelial growth factor stimulates collateral developments in vivo. *Lab Invest* 1996; **75:** 487–501.

12. Giordano FJ, Ping P, McKirnan MD et al. Intracoronary gene transfer of fibroblast growth factor-5 increases blood flow and contractile function in an ischemic region of the heart. *Nature Med* 1996; **2:** 534–9.

13. Nabel EG, Pompili VJ, Plautz GE, Nabel GJ. Gene transfer and vascular disease. *Cardiovasc Res* 1994; **28:** 445–55.

14. Rosenfeld MA, Yoshimura K, Trapnell BC et al. In vivo transfer of the human cystic fibrosis transmembrane conductance regulator gene to airway epithelium. *Cell* 1992; **68:** 143–55.

**164**

15. Yang Y, Nunes FA, Berencsi K et al. Cellular immunity to viral antigens limits E1-deleted adenoviruses for gene therapy. *Proc Natl Acad Sci USA* 1994; **91:** 4407–11.

16. Springer ML, Chen AS, Kraft PE et al. VEGF gene delivery to muscle: potential role for vasculogenesis in adults. *Mol Cell* 1998; **2:** 549–58.

17. Magovern CJ, Mack CA, Zhang J et al. Regional angiogenesis induced in non-ischemic tissue by an adenoviral vector expressing vascular endothelial growth factor. *Hum Gene Ther* 1997; **8:** 215–27.

18. Mack CA, Magovern CJ, Budenbender KT et al. Salvage angiogenesis induced by adenoviral-mediated gene transfer of vascular endothelial growth factor protects against ischemic vascular occlusion. *J Vasc Surg* 1998; **27:** 699–709.

19. Magovern CJ, Mack CA, Zhang J et al. Direct in vivo gene transfer to canine myocardium using a replication-deficient adenovirus vector. *Ann Thorac Surg* 1996; **62:** 425–34.

20. Mack CA, Patel SR, Schwarz EA et al. Biological bypass utilizing adenovirus-mediated gene transfer of the cDNA for vascular endothelial growth factor 121 improves myocardial perfusion and function in the ischemic porcine heart. *J Thorac Cardiovasc Surg* 1998; **115:** 168–77.

21. Patel SR, Lee LY, Mack CA et al. Safety of direct myocardial administration of an adenovirus vector coding for vascular endothelial growth factor 121. *Hum Gene Ther* 1999; **10:** 1331–48.

22. Rosengart TK, Lee LY, Patel SR. Angiogenesis gene therapy: phase I assessment of direct intramyocardial administration of an adenovirus vector expressing the VEGF121 cDNA to individuals with clinically significant severe coronary artery disease. *Circulation* 1999; **99** (in press).

# 13. Basic Fibroblast Growth Factor Protein for Peripheral Vascular Disease

Daisy F Lazarous

The principal treatment for atherosclerotic occlusive peripheral vascular disease (PVD) is surgical revascularization, since currently available medical therapies have not been consistently effective. A therapy aimed at increasing collateral growth or nature's own bypass vessels may be an option for patients with PVD. Such a novel method is the use of peptide growth factors like basic fibroblast growth factor (bFGF) and vascular endothelial growth factor (VEGF) to promote angiogenesis in ischemic lower extremity tissues. Preclinical experiments with both angiogenic peptides have led to the start of trials in patients with PVD. This chapter outlines the experimental studies of bFGF and briefly discusses the ongoing clinical study in patients with intermittent claudication.

## Basic fibroblast growth factor (bFGF)

bFGF (or FGF2) is one of the best characterized of the fibroblast growth factor family of polypeptides,[1] and is a potent angiogenic agent both in vitro and in vivo. It has a molecular weight of 18 kDa and is a non-secreted, heparin-binding polypeptide that is mitogenic for a variety of cell types. bFGF also acts as a differentiating factor, chemotactic agent, inducer of plasminogen activator, and/or metalloproteinase, depending on the target cell type.[2] bFGF interacts with low-affinity cell surface receptors (heparan sulfate proteoglycans in subendothelial matrix), as well as specific high-affinity tyrosine kinase receptors.[3]

The specific events responsible for the development of collaterals are complex, and the release and expression of several angiogenic growth factors has been postulated to play an important part. Exogenous growth factor could potentially accelerate and enhance the process of collateral development.

## Potential mechanisms of bFGF action

Ischemia (or a transcollateral pressure gradient, or both) is thought to be a primer for pharmacologically driven collateralization of ischemic tissues. There are experimental data to suggest that angiogenic peptides exert their maximal effect on collateral growth in the presence of active ischemia. Lazarous and colleagues[4] have shown that administration of bFGF, synchronized with the interval of maximum ischemia, enhanced myocardial angiogenesis and collateral perfusion. Additional treatment beyond the period of ischemia did not elicit further collateral development.[5] Yang and colleagues[6] found that heparin exerted an angiogenic effect in a rat femoral artery ligation model in the presence (but not in the absence) of exercise. While exercise may have a direct effect on collateral development, its role in inducing ischemia – which then facilitates the action of bFGF – may be a far more important factor in stimulating angiogenesis.

## Animal models of hindlimb ischemia

bFGF has been extensively studied in animal models of myocardial angiogenesis, and less so in hindlimb ischemia. The salient preclinical studies of the effects of bFGF on collateral growth in animal models of hindlimb ischemia have been performed in rabbits (Figure 13.1)[7,8] and rats.[9,10] bFGF has been studied by different routes, including intra-arterial infusion, intravenous bolus administration or infusion, and intramuscular and subcutaneous injections into the ischemic muscle bed. Intravenous bolus bFGF may be ineffective in inducing angiogenesis,[11] probably because of first pass lung uptake by low affinity receptors.[12] bFGF tissue deposition is concentration-dependent, in that there is maximal uptake at the point of delivery where the intravascular concentration is highest, which favours intra-arterial delivery into the vascular territory of the ischemic bed.

In a rat ischemic hindlimb model, continuous intravenous bFGF promoted collateralization. bFGF (1 μg/day) was infused into the femoral artery over 2 weeks after experimentally induced femoral artery occlusion.[10] One week of intravenous bFGF infusion produced an intermediate improvement in blood flow compared with placebo, with marked improvement after 2 weeks of bFGF infusion and no further change after infusion for 4 weeks. There was increased calf muscle blood flow as measured with radiolabeled microspheres, increased muscle capillary density, expansion of upper thigh collateral vessels, and enhanced muscle performance during nerve stimulation. Interestingly, the efficacy of bFGF was dependent on the duration of therapy, suggesting again that the amount of bFGF reaching the target tissue is limited after intravenous delivery. In another rat hindlimb model, hindlimb ischemia was induced surgically by ligation of the distal external iliac and femoral arteries. Implantation of heparin-sepharose pellets (controlled-release drug delivery system) containing bFGF (40 μg/kg) into the ischemic muscle resulted in improved hindlimb blood flow.[9]

**168**

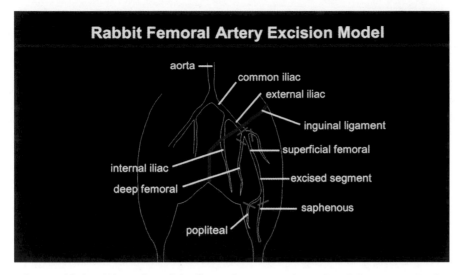

**Rabbit Femoral Artery Excision Model**

aorta — common iliac
external iliac
inguinal ligament
superficial femoral
internal iliac
deep femoral
excised segment
saphenous
popliteal

*Figure 13.1:* *All branches of the femoral artery are ligated and the common and superficial femoral arteries are excised from the inguinal ligament to just distal to the bifurcation into the popliteal and saphenous arteries.*

In rabbits, repeated intramuscular injections of 1 µg bFGF, or 3 µg bFGF daily for 2 weeks improved tissue perfusion and capillary density, and protected against skeletal muscle infarction.[15]

Heparin binds bFGF and stabilizes it against deactivation and proteolytic cleavage.[13] It is likely that tissue deposition and serum half life of bFGF would be altered by heparin, but the therapeutic implications of concomitant heparin and bFGF use are unclear at present.

Acidic fibroblast growth factor (aFGF, or FGF1) is an angiogenic factor that possesses 55% sequence homology with bFGF, and is not secreted by intact cells. A recent study investigated the aFGF/heparin regimen as a means of augmenting collateral vessel growth in a rat hindlimb ischemia model.[14] Daily subcutaneous injections of human recombinant aFGF protein with and without heparin (1 µg aFGF, 0.05 mg heparin) into the hindlimb region distal to the point of unilateral femoral artery ligation was done for 10 days immediately after vascular occlusion. The number of vessels assessed histologically in the skeletal muscle tissues distal to the vascular ligation, and mitogenic activity shown by the presence of proliferating cell nuclear antigen on immunohistochemical analysis, were increased. Heparin alone significantly accelerated angiogenesis, but the administration of aFGF with and without heparin resulted in a greater degree of improvement. bFGF and heparin increased blood flow, while protamine decreased collateral blood flow in a rat model of severe hindlimb ischemia.[9]

In a rabbit model, transposition of a muscle pedicle flap to an ischemic hindlimb has resulted in the development of new blood vessels that connect the arterial circulation of the flap to the circulation of the limb. bFGF infusion (3 ng/h) at the point of flap-muscle interface for 7 days via mini-osmotic pumps significantly augmented new blood vessel development.[15] Both bFGF and VEGF significantly promoted collateral vessel development in a dog model of femoral artery ligation.[16]

## Gene therapy experiments with FGF

Hypothesizing that a secreted gene product may be more effective than a non-secreted form, a recent study investigated arterial gene transfer of naked DNA encoding for aFGF, the non-secreted form, and a secreted form with a hydrophobic leader sequence. In rabbits, the plasmid encoding the secreted aFGF had more angiographically visible collaterals than either the control or the non-secreted form. Limb blood pressure and vascular resistance, both under basal conditions and after nitroprusside, as well as capillary density, were also superior in the secreted gene product group.[17]

## Clinical trial design

In designing clinical trials in PVD, selection of patients should take into account the known preclinical toxicity of bFGF.[18] Growth factors may increase the vascular supply of pre-existing tumors[19] or create angiomas.[20] Endothelial growth factors have been implicated as mediators of intraocular neovascularization[21] and retinal new blood vessel growth may occur. Neointimal proliferation may lead to restenosis. Growth factors like VEGF, which have endothelial cell specificity in vitro, may lose that specificity in vivo because of enhanced vascular permeability. This results in leaking of other mitogens like platelet derived growth factor, as well as attraction of monocytes to the site of vascular injury, leading to increased neointimal formation (Figure 13.2).[22] Angiogenesis inhibitors reduce plaque growth in animals,[23] and hence angiogenic agents may conceivably worsen atherosclerotic plaques. bFGF has the potential to induce a nephropathy with proteinuria at higher doses or with repeated administration over time.[18] Thus, diabetic retinopathy, cancer, and renal dysfunction should be considered as exclusion criteria. Another factor to be taken into consideration is the large placebo response that is common in PVD patients. In a review of 75 studies of medical therapies for PVD, 84% of the trials reported benefit if the design was

Neointima

Media

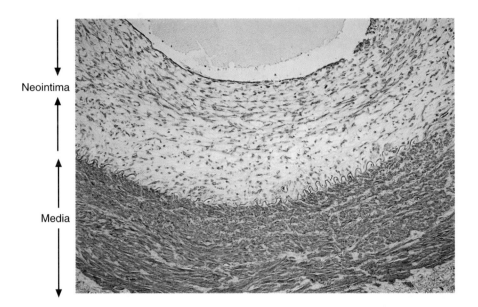

*Figure 13.2:* Neointima formation in response to injury in the iliac artery of an animal treated with VEGF protein. The predominant cell type in the neointima was smooth muscle cells, as identified by immunohistochemical staining for alpha smooth muscle actin (pink cells).

open or uncontrolled, whereas only 32% reported improvement if the design was placebo-controlled.[24] Thus, randomized, placebo-controlled trials are of paramount importance.

A clinical trial of bFGF in patients with intermittent claudication was recently done at the National Heart, Lung, and Blood Institute, Bethesda, MD, USA. This phase I double-blind, placebo-controlled, dose-escalation study assessed the safety and effects of bFGF on calf blood flow.[25] Preliminary data indicate that bFGF is safe in human beings and well tolerated. bFGF administered intra-arterially into the femoral artery of the ischemic leg significantly improved calf blood flow and reduced vascular resistance. This was accompanied by subjective improvement in symptoms in treated patients. These preliminary results in PVD patients are encouraging but not definitive, and a larger confirmatory phase II multicenter trial is planned in patients with intermittent claudication and critical limb ischemia (Scios Inc, Mountainview, CA).

PVD clinical trials with bFGF currently use improvement in exercise tolerance and functional outcomes as efficacy endpoints. It is important to delineate mechanistic insights for these improvements, such as correlative changes in blood flow and calf muscle metabolism. Angiography is an inadequate endpoint, because collateral vessels less than 200 μ in diameter (the size commonly induced by angiogenic therapy) are not visualized by this technique.

VEGF and bFGF exhibit synergism in vitro. In a rabbit model, combined administration of VEGF and bFGF stimulated significantly greater and more rapid augmentation of collateral circulation, resulting in superior hemodynamic improvement compared with either VEGF or bFGF alone.[8] This synergism will need to be explored further in patients with PVD.

## New frontiers in angiogenesis research

Exciting new frontiers are emerging in the field of angiogenesis. Recent findings suggest that putative endothelial cell progenitors or angioblasts incorporate into sites of active angiogenesis, suggesting that this approach may be useful to augment collateral vessel growth to ischemic tissues and as a delivery means for anti- or pro-angiogenic agents.[26] Discovery of the angiopoietin/Tie2 receptor pathways will probably open up new areas of research. Angiopoietin-1 is an angiogenic factor that signals through the endothelial cell-specific Tie2 receptor tyrosine kinase. Angiopoietin-2 is a naturally occurring antagonist for Ang1 and Tie2.[27] Also, recent data suggest that monocyte accumulation and activation may play an important part in angiogenesis and collateral growth.[28]

In summary, preclinical studies are a compelling argument for a potential salutary role of FGFs in clinical syndromes of hindlimb ischemia. Early clinical observations seem to suggest that such benefit may be possible in patients with intermittent claudication. In planning clinical angiogenesis trials in PVD, the optimal agent or combination of agents, best mode of drug delivery, and dosage need to be identified. Delivery of the gene may not be a requisite, since recent data in animals[29] and preliminary data in human beings[25] suggest that one or two doses of recombinant bFGF may be sufficient.

## References

1. Gospodarowicz D. Fibroblast growth factor. *Crit Rev Oncog* 1989; **1:** 1–26.

2. Sato Y, Rifkin DB. Autocrine activities of basic fibroblast growth factor: regulation of endothelial cell movement, plasminogen activator synthesis, and DNA synthesis. *J Cell Biol* 1988; **107:** 1199–205.

3. Bashkin P, Doctrow S, Klagsbrun M et al. Basic fibroblast growth factor binds to subendothelial extracellular matrix and is released by heparitinase and heparin-like molecules. *Biochemistry* 1989; **28:** 1737–43.

4. Lazarous DF, Scheinowitz M, Shou M et al. Effects of chronic systemic administration of basic fibroblast growth factor on collateral development in the canine heart. *Circulation* 1995; **91:** 145–53.

5. Shou M, Thirumurti V, Rajanayagam MAS et al. Effect of basic fibroblast growth factor on myocardial angiogenesis in dogs with mature collateral vessels. *J Am Coll Cardiol* 1997; **29:** 1102–6.

6. Yang HT, Ogilvie RW, Terjung RL. Heparin increases exercise-induced collateral blood flow in rats with femoral artery ligation. *Circ Res* 1995; **76:** 448–56.

7. Baffour R, Berman J, Garb JL et al. Enhanced angiogenesis and growth of collaterals by *in vivo* administration of basic fibroblast growth factor in a rabbit model of acute lower limb ischemia: dose-response effect of basic fibroblast growth factor. *J Vasc Surg* 1992; **161:** 181–91.

8. Asahara T, Bauters C, Zheng LP et al. Synergistic effect of vascular endothelial growth factor and basic fibroblast growth factor on angiogenesis in vivo. *Circulation* 1995; II-365–71.

9. Chleboun JO, Martins RN. The development and enhancement of the collateral circulation in an animal model of lower limb ischemia. *Aust N Z J Surg* 1994; **64:** 202–7.

10. Yang HT, Deschenes MR, Ogilvie RW, Terjung RT. Basic fibroblast growth factor increases collateral blood flow in rats with femoral artery ligation. *Circ Res* 1996; **79:** 62–9.

11. Thirumurti V, Shou M, Hodge E et al. Lack of efficacy of intravenous basic fibroblast growth factor in promoting myocardial angiogenesis. *J Am Coll Cardiol* 1998; **31** (suppl A): 801–6.

12. Lazarous DF, Shou M, Stiber JA et al. Pharmacodynamics of basic fibroblast growth factor: route of administration determines myocardial and systemic distribution. *Cardiovasc Res* 1997; **36:** 78–85.

13. Roghani M, Mansukhani A, Dell'Era P et al. Heparin increases the affinity of basic fibroblast growth factor for its receptor but is not required for binding. *J Biol Chem* 1994; **269:** 3976–84.

14. Rosengart TK, Budenbender KT, Duenas M et al. Therapeutic angiogenesis: a comparative study of the angiogenic potential of acidic fibroblast growth factor and heparin. *J Vasc Surg* 1997; **26:** 302–12.

15. Bush RL, Pevec WC, Ndoye A et al. Regulation of new blood vessel growth into ischemic skeletal muscle. *J Vasc Surg* 1998; **28:** 919–28.

16. Ibukiyama C. Angiogenic therapy using fibroblast growth factors and vascular endothelial growth factors for ischemic vascular lesions. *Jpn Heart J* 1996; **37:** 285–300.

17. Tabata H, Silver M, Isner JM. Arterial gene transfer of acidic fibroblast growth

factor for therapeutic angiogenesis in vivo: critical role of secretion signal in use of naked DNA. *Cardiovasc Res* 1997; **35**: 470–9.

18. Mazué G, Newman AJ, Scampini G et al. The histopathology of kidney changes in rats and monkeys following intravenous administration of massive doses of FCE 26184, human basic fibroblast growth factor. *Toxicol Pathol* 1993; **21**: 490–501.

19. Folkman J. Fighting cancer by attacking its blood supply. *Sci Am* 1996; **275**: 150–4.

20. Schwarz ER, Spealman MT, Patterson M et al. Effect of intra myocardial injection of DNA expressing vascular endothelial growth factor in myocardial infarct tissue in the rat heart – angiogenesis and angioma formation. *Circulation* 1998; **456** (suppl 1): 2397.

21. Aiello LP, Pierce EA, Foley ED et al. Suppression of retinal neovascularization in vivo by inhibition of vascular endothelial growth factor (VEGF) using soluble VEGF-receptor chimeric proteins. *Proc Natl Acad Sci* USA 1995; **92**: 10457–61.

22. Lazarous DF, Shou M, Scheinowitz M et al. Comparative effects of basic fibroblast growth factor and vascular endothelial growth factor on coronary collateral development and the arterial response to injury. *Circulation* 1996; **94**: 1074–82.

23. Moulton KS, Heller E, Konerding MA et al. Angiogenesis inhibitors reduce plaque growth. *Circulation* 1998; **454** (suppl 1): 2391.

24. Cameron HA, Waller PC, Ramsay LE. Drug treatment of intermittent claudication: a critical analysis of the methods and findings of published clinical trials, 1965–1985. *Br J Clin Pharmacol* 1988; **26**: 569–76.

25. Lazarous DF, Unger EF, Epstein SE et al. Effect of basic fibroblast growth factor on lower extremity blood flow in patients with intermittent claudication: preliminary results. *Circulation* 1998; **456** (suppl 1): 2398.

26. van der Zee R, Li T, Witzenbichler B et tal. Isolation of putative progenitor endothelial cells for angiogenesis. *Science* 1997; **275**: 964–7.

27. Papadopoulos N, Daly TJ, Davis S et al. Angiopoietin-2, a natural antagonist for Tie2 that disrupts in vivo angiogenesis. *Science* 1997; **277**: 55–60.

28. Arras M, Ito WD, Scholz D et al. Monocyte activation in angiogenesis and collateral growth in the rabbit hind limb. *J Clin Invest* 1998; **101**: 40–50.

29. Rajanayagam S, Shou M, Thirumurti V et al. Two intracoronary doses of basic fibroblast growth factor enhance collateral blood flow in dogs. *J Am Coll Cardiol* 1996; **27** (suppl A): 36A.

# 14. Basic Fibroblast Growth Factor Protein for Coronary Artery Disease

Roger J Laham and Michael Simons

## Introduction

Ischemic heart disease remains the leading cause of death in the developed world. Cardiovascular disease claimed 960 592 lives in 1995 (in the USA, 41.5% of all deaths) with 1 100 000 new and recurrent cases of acute coronary syndromes per year and 13 900 000 people alive today (USA) having a history of myocardial infarction or angina pectoris. Current therapeutic approaches aim to relieve symptoms and cardiac events by reducing myocardial oxygen demand with medical therapy, preventing further disease progression by modifying risk factors, or restoring flow to a localized segment of the arterial tree by coronary angioplasty (PTCA) or bypass surgery (CABG).[1] However, it is becoming increasingly clear that a significant number of patients with ischemic heart disease are not candidates for PTCA/CABG or have incomplete revascularization with these procedures.[1] In fact, up to 20–37% of patients with ischemic heart disease either cannot undergo CABG or PTCA or receive incomplete revascularization with these standard revascularization strategies.[1–3] Many of these patients have residual symptoms or myocardial ischemia despite maximal medical therapy. Therefore, an alternative revascularization strategy is required in these patients to relieve angina and to improve myocardial ischemia. Therapeutic angiogenesis may serve this purpose by providing new venues for blood flow.[1,3–5]

Normal myocardium lacks native collateral vessels, but prolonged or recurrent myocardial ischemia can initiate the formation of a plexus of collateral vessels in zones of ischemic myocardium.[6–11] However, while these collateral channels can serve to "revascularize" ischemic myocardium, the high requirement for surgical and percutaneous revascularization procedures each year in the USA (400 000 CABG, 600 000 PTCA) attests to the fact that native collateral vessel formation is frequently insufficient to compensate for the diminished blood flow that results from coronary artery disease.[6–11] The rapid development of growth factor therapy in patients with advanced ischemic heart disease over the past 5 years offers hope of a new treatment strategy based on generation of new blood supply in the diseased heart.[1,12–15] Several growth factors, including the fibroblast growth factor (FGF) family, vascular endothelial growth factor (VEGF) family, platelet derived growth (PDGF) family, angiopoietins, cytokines such as I1-6 and I1-8, "master switch" genes such as hypoxia-inducible factor (HIF)-1α and molecules such as nitric oxide (NO), platelet activating factor (PAF), and substance P all stimulate blood vessel growth under different circumstances.[1,3,12,16,17]

## Mechanism of growth factor induced angiogenesis

Angiogenesis is a complex process that involves stimulation of endothelial cell proliferation and migration, stimulation of extracellular matrix breakdown, attraction of pericytes and macrophages, stimulation of smooth muscle cell proliferation and migration, formation and "sealing" of new vascular structures, and deposition of new matrix.[1,12,16] It is likely that coordinated action of several mitogens and cascades is needed to achieve this process.

The ability of growth factors such as basic fibroblast growth factor (bFGF) to increase the rate of endothelial cell proliferation has been shown in several animal studies.[18–20] Interestingly, in the setting of regional myocardial ischemia, endothelial cell proliferation rate is largely limited to the ischemic zone even during systemic (or non-selective coronary) growth factor administration.[18,20–22] Similarly, in the setting of arterial injury, endothelial cell growth is limited to the immediate surrounding area and not the entire vascular tree.[19] It is apparent, therefore, that potent local factors, including perhaps angiogenesis promoters and inhibitors, control the local angiogenic response. In addition, limited expression of high affinity growth factor receptors such as FGF R1, flk-1, and flt-1 may limit the angiogenic potency of these cytokines in normal tissues.[23–25]

In addition to direct stimulation of endothelial cell growth, all growth factors possess a wide spectrum of biological activities that may be involved in angiogenic response. Particularly interesting and important may be the ability to stimulate production of NO.[26–28] Another intriguing and poorly understood feature of angiogenic growth factor therapy is the occurrence of an extensive response (in terms of neovascularization) 3–4 weeks after a singe bolus growth factor administration.[1,29,30] Since no known pharmacokinetic profile can explain this effect, and since the half life of most growth factors is far shorter than the time span before their biological activity becomes observable, one is left with speculation either that there is a prolonged retention of the growth factors in ischemic tissues secondary, perhaps, to heparan sulfate binding, or that the single bolus administration sets of a positive feedback loop that functions over the ensuing weeks.

Therapeutic administration of either FGFs or VEGF results in both intramyocardial as well as epicardial neovascularization. The relative importance of these events is not clear, however. The process of intramyocardial collateral development (angiogenesis) is characterized by the appearance of thin walled vessels with a poorly developed tunica media that are under 200 μm in diameter, and by an increase in the number of true capillaries (<20 μm in diameter containing only a single endothelial layer). Neo-arteriogenesis, on the other hand, is characterized by development of larger vessels (>200 μm in diameter) with well developed media and adventitia, that usually form close to the site of the occlusion of a major epicardial coronary artery (bridging collaterals) or extend from one coronary artery to another (Figure 14.1).[3,17] The distinction between these two groups of newly formed vessels is important because of their location, but also because stimuli for their development appear to be quite different and because they show different physiological properties. Although increased intramyocardial vessel growth may promote better distribution of flow throughout the ischemic myocardium, epicardial collateral development may well be necessary to provide the source of blood flow to intramyocardial vessels that is impaired by obstruction of native epicardial vessels. It is not known whether both of these processes respond to the same stimuli, although it seems clear that ischemia is far more important in stimulation of intramyocardial than epicardial collateral development. Furthermore, although angiographic and

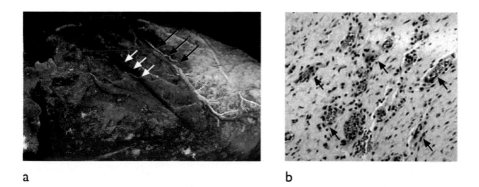

a
b

***Figure 14.1:*** *(a) Coronary casting of a porcine ameroid constrictor model heart with injection of blue polymer in the left circumflex artery (LCX), red polymer in the left anterior descending artery (LAD), and white polymer in the right coronary artery (RCA), followed by digestion of the myocardium by KOH. Note large epicardial collateral vessel from the LAD to LCX distribution (closed arrows) and a large epicardial collateral with inflow from both LAD and RCA distributions to the LCX (open arrows). (b) Histological section of ischemic myocardium treated with bFGF shows an increased number of capillaries (arrows). Many of these small blood vessels are lined by endothelial cells with large, hyperchromatic nuclei, suggesting new vascular in-growth.*

**177**

morphometric studies show that both FGFs and VEGF augment both the presence of epicardial collaterals and intramyocardial neovascularization, it is not clear if these modes of new vessel growth are in any way growth-factor specific. On theoretical grounds, FGFs may be more likely to induce neo-arteriogenesis and VEGF angiogenesis, but the cross-talk between various components of angiogenic response and the ability of bFGF to induce VEGF expression[31] suggests that there may be little difference in the final result.

## Basic fibroblast growth factor

Basic fibroblast growth factor, otherwise known as bFGF or FGF2, was the second discovered member of the fibroblast growth factor family, which now comprises more than 22 different fibroblast growth factors.[1,3,17] bFGF belongs to a family of structurally related polypeptides, characterized by high affinity to heparin and heparan sulfate. bFGF is a 16.5 kD 146 aminoacid protein that binds with high affinity ($10^{-11}$ M) to specific tyrosine kinase receptors, and with lower affinity ($10^{-9}$ M) to cellular heparan sulfates. It has anti-apoptotic effects and is a potent mitogen for cells of mesenchymal, neural, and epithelial origin.[15,32–34] In particular, bFGF is a powerful angiogenic agent, both in vitro and in vivo, owing to its proliferative effects on vascular endothelial cells.[1,35,36]

bFGF is indeed the most extensively studied growth factor in a variety of angiogenesis models. bFGF is detectable in both atrial and ventricular adult myocardium, as well as in intramyocardial vessels.[37] Homozygous delition of the bFGF gene is not associated with any significant phenotype except for decreased vascular smooth muscle contractility, low blood pressure, and thrombocytosis.[38]

## Pre-clinical evaluation

The ability of FGF2 to induce significant angiogenesis in mature tissues was suggested by studies in canine and porcine infarction models. In these experiments, intracoronary injections of bFGF in the setting of acute coronary thrombosis in dogs, or intracoronary injections of 75–150 µg FGF2 containing affigel beads in pigs, led to significantly higher vessel count compared with controls.[39,40]

Studies of the therapeutic efficacy of bFGF in chronic myocardial ischemia have explored a variety of routes of administration in both canine and porcine models. The prototype for chronic myocardial ischemia has been the ameroid constrictor model, whereby an ameroid constrictor is placed around the left circumflex artery or the left anterior descending artery. The ameroid constrictor leads to gradual narrowing of the instrumented artery, which occludes completely over a

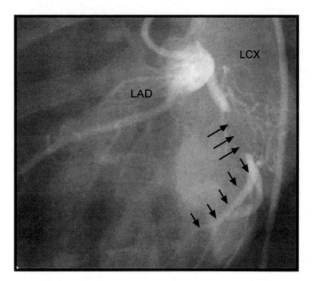

**Figure 14.2:** *Ameroid constrictor model: ameroid constrictor matched to artery diameter is placed on the left circumflex artery (LCX). Angiography 3 weeks post-implantation shows total occlusion of the LCX (black arrows) with faint filling of the distal circumflex artery (black arrows) by epicardial and intramyocardial collaterals.*

period of 3 to 4 weeks. The gradual occlusion, together with the formation of native collateral vessels, leads to chronic myocardial ischemia/myocardial hybernation with only limited subendocardial infarction (Figure 14.2). Daily injections of 110 μg bFGF for 18 days directly into the circumflex coronary artery distal to an ameroid occluder hastened restoration of flow in the compromised territory compared with normal saline controls.[41] Morphometric analysis of LCX myocardium showed equal capillary densities in both bFGF-treated and control animals, but a significant (2-fold) increase in the number of larger (>20 μm) vessels.[41] To examine the effect of systemic bFGF administration, the same group of investigators carried out daily left atrial injections of 1.74 mg of bFGF for 18 days. This mode of bFGF administration resulted in early augmentation of coronary flow in the growth factor-treated animals that was similar to that seen with direct intracoronary injections but was lost by day 38.[42,43] Prolonged (up to 6 months) infusions of bFGF did not result in any further increase in collateral blood flow, which was identical in bFGF and saline-treated animals – underscoring the priming role of ischemia of bFGF-induced collateral development.[44] The myocardial angiogenic effect of bFGF was not associated with structural or vasoproliferative effect on the non-ischemic retina of dogs with myocardial ischemia.[45] In the same canine model, 7-day systemic arterial administration of bFGF enhanced collateral development without increasing neointimal accumulation at sites of vascular injury.[43]

In summary, these studies clearly showed increased coronary perfusion after bFGF treatment that is probably predominantly mediated by neoarteriogenesis, as suggested by the lack of increase in capillary density.

Local perivascular delivery of bFGF was assessed in a porcine model of chronic myocardial ischemia (LCX ameroid occlusion). Heparin-alginate microcapsules were used for sustained delivery of bFGF. This form of delivery is characterized by first order release kinetics of growth factor from the polymer over a 4–5 week period, ease of implantation, and the absence of any inflammatory reaction associated with polymer placement.[19,46–49] Furthermore, perivascular delivery has a potential advantage of bypassing the endothelial barrier and avoiding rapid washout of growth factor due to rapid arterial blood flow.[50] Animals implanted with heparin-alginate pellets containing 8 µg bFGF at the time of ameroid placement (~5 µg released over the course of the experiment – about 328-fold less than previously discussed studies) showed significantly better preservation of perfusion of the ischemic zone during pacing compared with control animals.[48] In addition, ventricular function studies showed better preservation of regional left ventricular function in the ameroid-compromised territory at rest, and faster recovery after pacing in bFGF-treated animals. However, rapid pacing induced equal and significant deterioration in both bFGF-treated and control groups. Examination of the effect of progressively larger amounts of bFGF (10 and 100 µg) delivered in a similar manner in a pig model[46,47] showed substantial improvement in resting coronary blood flow in the chronically ischemic myocardium in both bFGF groups compared with controls, and gave an increase in angiographic collaterals.[47,48]

Analysis of left ventricular function showed a higher ejection fraction at rest and during pacing in both 10 and 100 µg bFGF groups compared with controls. Similarly, regional wall motion in the ischemic territory was better preserved at rest in both bFGF groups, although during rapid pacing only the 100 µg bFGF group maintained normal wall thickening.[47] Thus, perivascular sustained release FGF-2 resulted in a dose-dependent improvement of coronary perfusion accompanied by an improvement in left ventricular function.

Given this increase in the number of epicardial collaterals, the observed improvement in coronary blood flow and left ventricular function in these studies may equally have been due to bFGF-induced neoarteriogenesis and true myocardial angiogenesis. In addition to improving angiographic collaterals, myocardial perfusion, and left ventricular function, perivascular delivery of bFGF resulted in normalization of ischemia-induced impairment of endothelium-dependent vasodilation in the LCX ischemic area.[51] Additional studies of bFGF delivery methods showed enhanced new epicardial small-vessel growth following

**180**

intrapericardial space using an osmotic pump in a rabbit model of angiotensin-II induced left ventricular hypertrophy.[52]

Most attempts to stimulate myocardial angiogenesis have employed methods of prolonged growth factor delivery. However, some of these options, such as repeated intracardiac injections or infusions, are either unfeasible or impractical in patients with ischemic heart disease. Therefore, single dose delivery (either intracoronary, intravenous, or intrapericardial) was attempted. Intrapericardial delivery of bFGF (30 µg up to 2 mg) in a porcine LCX ameroid occlusion model resulted in significant increases in left-to-left angiographic collaterals and blood flow, accompanied by improvements in MR measured myocardial perfusion and function in the ischemic territory, and by histological evidence of increased myocardial vascularity.[53] None of these benefits was seen in saline- or heparin-treated ischemic animals.

Local intramyocardial injection of bFGF 4–5 weeks after creation of an infarct in pigs resulted in an increase in the number of arterioles but not capillaries compared with controls.[54] bFGF's effect was potentiated by co-administration with heparin.

In addition to stimulation of neovascularization in the setting of chronic ischemia, bFGF administration also has beneficial effects in acute myocardial ischemia. Intracoronary administration of 20 µg bFGF in a canine experimental myocardial infarct model improved cardiac systolic function, reduced infarct size, and increased the number of arterioles and capillaries in the infarct zone.[39] Similar findings were observed with intrapericardial injection of 30 µg bFGF in dogs with acute myocardial infarction, which resulted in significant reduction in the size of myocardial infarction and improvement in left ventricular function, both of which were augmented by a simultaneous administration of heparan sulfate.[55] These findings were duplicated in an acute ischemia/reperfusion study in which 10 µg bFGF 10 min after initiation of coronary occlusion and again immediately before reperfusion resulted in significant salvage of myocardium at risk compared with control animals.[56] These beneficial effects may have resulted from the vasodilatory action of bFGF-2,[57,58] a myocardial protective effect, possibly via a nitric-oxide-dependent pathway,[59] as well as an anti-apoptic effect.[60,61]

## Clinical evaluation

There is a large number of patients with ischemic heart disease who are suboptimal candidates for coronary artery bypass surgery or angioplasty, and there is a relatively high percentage of patients undergoing CABG with incomplete revascularization. The studies described above, with their promising preclinical results of bFGF induced angiogenesis, propelled the use of these

**181**

growth factors in clinical studies of therapeutic angiogenesis. To date, few studies have been published, but several studies using bFGF are currently testing the therapeutic potential of growth factors in ischemic heart disease.[1,4]

An NIH-sponsored double-blind placebo-controlled trial is examining the effect of local perivascular bFGF (10 µg or 100 µg) delivered using heparin-alginate beads implanted at the time of coronary artery bypass surgery in patients who have a viable but underperfused myocardial territory that is not amenable to bypass grafting. Growth factor-containing bead implantation added on average $2.8 \pm 1.1$ min to operative time. Interim analysis of the first 24 patients showed no acute or chronic hemodynamic effects following growth factor implantation, and no significant changes in hematology or chemistry profiles during follow-up; no other adverse events were noted.[4,62,63] Plasma bFGF concentrations did not increase above baseline. Nuclear perfusion scans and MRI determined target regional wall motion and target wall perfusion showed improved results with administration of 100 µg bFGF.[4,63]

A phase I dose-escalation study of intracoronary (52 patients) and intravenous (14 patients) bFGF in patients with severe coronary disease has been completed and showed the safety and tolerability of bFGF. The doses tested ranged from 0.33 µg/kg (ideal bodyweight) to 48 µg/kg. Hypotension occurred at 48 µg/kg in two of ten patients in that group and was successfully treated with intravenous fluids. The maximum tolerated dose was 36 µg/kg (defined by hypotension). There were no changes in ECG or cardiac enzymes and no peripheral or pulmonary oedema. Transient leukocytosis was noted on day 2 at doses of 24 µg/kg or more, and transient proteinuria was observed in five of 66 patients and was not dose-related. No retinal toxicity was observed at 60 days.[64] The preliminary efficacy data is promising, with improved exercise time, improved quality of life (Seattle Angina Questionnaire), and improved target wall motion and perfusion using magnetic resonance imaging.[64] This, however, was an uncontrolled study in a patient population with a known placebo effect. The phase II study is currently underway.

A phase I double-blind, placebo-controlled, dose-escalation study of intra-arterial bFGF in patients with intermittent claudication has also been done. Patients were randomly assigned placebo (n = 6), 10 µg/kg bFGF (n = 4), 30 µg/kg bFGF once (n = 5), and 30 µg/kg bFGF twice (n = 4). The study drug was infused into the femoral artery of the ischemic leg. Calf blood flow was measured with strain-gauge plethysmography in the final two treated groups and in four patients on placebo, prior to treatment, and at 1 month and 6 months after treatment. Intra-arterial bFGF was well tolerated, and improved calf blood flow at 1 month by 66 $\pm$26% (mean $\pm$ SEM), and at 6 months by 153 $\pm$ 51% (n = 9, p = 0.002) The magnitude of increase in calf blood flow was greater in patients who received two doses of bFGF than in those who had one dose of 30 µg/kg. Flow did not change significantly in the placebo group.

**182**

# References

1.  Laham R, Simons M. Therapeutic angiogenesis in myocardial ischemia. In: *Angiogenesis and Cardiovascular Disease*. Simons WA (ed.). Oxford University Press, 1999.

2.  Jones EL, Craver JM, Guyton RA et al. Importance of complete revascularization in performance of the coronay bypass operation. *Am J Cardiol* 1983; **51:** 7–12.

3.  Schaper W, Ito W. Molecular mechanisms of collateral vessel growth. *Circ Res* 1996; **79:** 911–19.

4.  Sellke FW, Laham RJ, Edelman ER et al. Therapeutic angiogenesis with basic fibroblast growth factor: technique and early results. *Ann Thorac Surg* 1998; **65:** 1540–4.

5.  Schumacher B, Pecher P, von Specht B, Stegmann T. Induction of neoangiogenesis in ischemic myocardium by human growth factors. *Circulation* 1998; **97:** 645–50.

6.  Chilian WM, Mass HJ, Williams SE et al. Microvascular occlusions promote coronary collateral growth. *Am J Physiol* 1990; **258:** H1103–11.

7.  Fujita M, Sasayama S, Asanoi H et al. Improvement of treadmill capacity and collateral circulation as a result of exercise with heparin pretreatment in patients with effort angina. *Circulation* 1988; **77:** 1022–9.

8.  Iosseliani DG, Koval AN, Bhattacharya PK. Myocardial perfusion in new-onset angina patients with single vessel disease. *Int J Card Imaging* 1994; **10:** 155–9.

9.  Nishigami K, Ando M, Hayasaki K. Effects of antecedent anginal episodes and coronary artery stenosis on left ventricular function during coronary occlusion. *Am Heart J* 1995; **130:** 244–7.

10. Noma M, Tomoike H, Ando H et al. Collateral development induced by repetitive brief coronary occlusion relates to the functional state of pre-existing collateral. *Jpn Circ J* 1994; **58:** 269–77.

11. Sabri MN, DiSciascio G, Cowley MJ et al. Coronary collateral recruitment: functional significance and relation to rate of vessel closure. *Am Heart J* 1991, **121:** 876–80.

12. Ware JA, Simons M. Angiogenesis in ischemic heart disease. *Nature Med* 1997; **3:** 158–64.

13. Isner JM, Feldman LJ. Gene therapy for arterial disease. *Lancet* 1994; **344:** 1653–4.

14. Unger EF, Shou M, Sheffield CD et al. Extracardiac to coronary anastomoses support regional left ventricular function in dogs. *Am J Physiol* 1993; **264:** H1567–74.

15. Folkman J. Angiogenic therapy of human heart. *Circulation* 1998; **97:** 628–9.

16. Simons M, Ware JA. Food for starving hearts. *Nature Med* 1996; **2**: 519–20.

17. Schaper W. Collateral vessel growth in the human heart: role of fibroblast growth factor-2. *Circulation* 1996; **94**: 600–1.

18. Muhlhauser J, Pili R, Merrill JJ et al. In vivo angiogenesis induced by recombinant adenovirus vectors coding either for secreted or nonsecreted forms of acidic fibroblast growth factor. *Hum Gene Ther* 1995; **6**: 1457–65.

19. Edelman ER, Nugent MA, Smith LT, Karnovsky MJ. Basic fibroblast growth factor enhances the coupling of intimal hyperplasia and proliferation of vasa vasorum in injured rat arteries. *J Clin Invest* 1992; **89**: 465–73.

20. Seghezzi G, Patel S, Ren CJ et al. Fibroblast growth factor-2 (FGF-2) induces vascular endothelial growth factor (VEGF) expression in the endothelial cells of forming capillaries: an autocrine mechanism contributing to angiogenesis. *J Cell Biol* 1999; **141**: 1659–73.

21. Kuwabara K, Ogawa S, Matsumoto M et al. Hypoxia-mediated induction of acidic/basic fibroblast growth factor and platelet-derived growth factor in mononuclear phagocytes stimulates growth of hypoxic endothelial cells. *Proc Natl Acad Sci USA* 1995; **92**: 4606–10.

22. Lindner V, Majack RA, Reidy MA. Basic fibroblast growth factor stimulates endothelial regrowth and proliferation in denuded arteries. *J Clin Invest* 1990; **85**: 2004–8.

23. Gonzalez AM, Hill DJ, Logan A et al. Distribution of fibroblast growth factor (FGF)-2 and FGF receptor-1 messenger RNA expression and protein presence in the mid-trimester human fetus. *Pediatr Res* 1996; **39**: 375–85.

24. Jouanneau J, Plouet J, Moens G, Thiery JP. FGF-2 and FGF-1 expressed in rat bladder carcinoma cells have similar angiogenic potential but different tumorigenic properties in vivo. *Oncogene* 1997; **14**: 671–6.

25. Miao HQ, Ornitz DM, Aingorn E et al. Modulation of fibroblast growth factor-2 receptor binding, dimerization, signalling, and angiogenic activity by a synthetic heparin-mimicking polyanionic compound. *J Clin Invest* 1997; **99**: 1565–75.

26. Bastaki M, Nelli EE, Dell'Era P et al. Basic fibroblast growth factor-induced angiogenic phenotype in mouse endothelium: a study of aortic and microvascular endothelial cell lines. *Arterioscler Thromb Vasc Biol* 1997; **17**: 454–64.

27. Unthank JL, Nixon JC, Dalsing MC. Inhibition of NO synthase prevents acute collateral artery dilation in the rat hindlimb. *J Surg Res* 1996; **61**: 463–8.

28. Sellke FW, Wang SY, Stamler A et al. Enhanced microvascular relaxations to VEGF and bFGF in chronically ischemic porcine myocardium. *Am J Physiol* 1996; **271**: H713–20.

29. Lopez JJ, Laham RJ, Stamler A et al. VEGF administration in chronic myocardial ischemia in pigs. *Cardiovasc Res* 1998; **40**: 272–81.

30. Laham RJ, Hung D, Simons M. Therapeutic myocardial angiogenesis using percutaneous intrapericardial drug delivery. *Clin Cardiol* 1999; **22** (suppl 1): I-6–9.

31. Stavri GT, Zachary IC, Baskerville PA et al. Basic fibroblast growth factor upregulates the expression of vascular endothelial growth factor in vascular smooth muscle cells: synergistic interaction with hypoxia. *Circulation* 1995; **92:** 11–14.

32. Folkman J, Shing Y. Angiogenesis. *J Biol Chem* 1992; **267:** 10931–4.

33. Folkman J. Angiogenesis and angiogenesis inhibition: an overview. *EXS* 1997; **79:** 1–8.

34. Burgess W, Maciag T. The heparin-binding growth factor family of proteins. *Ann Rev Biochem* 1989; **58:** 575–606.

35. Thompson C, Challoner P, Neiman P, Groudine M. Expression of the c-myb protooncogene during cellular proliferation. *Nature* 1986; **319:** 374–80.

36. Gospodarowicz D. Expression and control of vascular endothelial cells: proliferation and differentiation by fibroblast growth factors. *J Invest Dermatol* 1989; **93:** 39S–47S.

37. Kardami E, Fandrich RR. Basic fibroblast growth factor in atria and ventricles of the vertebrate heart. *J Cell Biol* 1989; **109:** 1865–75.

38. Zhou M, Sutliff RL, Paul RJ et al. Fibroblast growth factor 2 control of vascular tone. *Nature Med* 1998; **4:** 201–7.

39. Yanagisawa-Miwa A, Uchida Y, Nakamura F et al. Salvage of infarcted myocardium by angiogenic action of basic fibroblast growth factor. *Science* 1992; **257:** 1401–3.

40. Battler A, Scheinowitz M, Bor A et al. Intracoronary injection of basic fibroblast growth factor enhances angiogenesis in infarcted swine myocardium. *J Am Coll Cardiol* 1993; **22:** 2001–6.

41. Unger EF, Banai S, Shou M et al. Basic fibroblast growth factor enhances myocardial collateral flow in a canine model. *Am J Physiol* 1994; **266:** H1588–95.

42. Lazarous DF, Scheinowitz M, Shou M et al. Effects of chronic systemic administration of basic fibroblast growth factor on collateral development in the canine heart. *Circulation* 1995; **91:** 145–53.

43. Lazarous DF, Shou M, Scheinowitz M et al. Comparative effects of basic fibroblast growth factor and vascular endothelial growth factor on coronary collateral development and the arterial response to injury. *Circulation* 1996; **94:** 1074–82.

44. Shou M, Thirumurti V, Rajanayagam S et al. Effect of basic fibroblast growth factor on myocardial angiogenesis in dogs with mature collateral vessels. *J Am Coll Cardiol* 1997; **29:** 1102–6.

45. Jacot JL, Laver NM, Glover JP et al. Histological evaluation of the canine retinal vasculature following chronic systemic administration of basic fibroblast growth factor. *J Anat* 1996; **188:** 349–54.

**185**

46. Lopez J, Edelman E, Stamler A et al. Local perivascular administration of basic fibroblast growth factor: drug delivery and toxicological evaluation. *Drug Metab Disposition* 1996; **24:** 922–4.

47. Lopez JJ, Edelman ER, Stamler A et al. Basic fibroblast growth factor in a porcine model of chronic myocardial ischemia: a comparison of angiographic, echocardiographic and coronary flow parameters. *J Pharmacol Exp Ther* 1997; **282:** 385–90.

48. Harada K, Grossman W, Friedman M et al. Basic fibroblast growth factor improves myocardial function in chronically ischemic porcine hearts. *J Clin Invest* 1994; **94:** 623–30.

49. Edelman ER, Mathiowitz E, Langer R, Klagsbrun M. Controlled and modulated release of basic fibroblast growth factor. *Biomaterials* 1991; **12:** 619–26.

50. Edelman ER, Nugent MA, Karnovsky MJ. Perivascular and intravenous administration of basic fibroblast growth factor: vascular and solid organ deposition. *Proc Natl Acad Sci USA* 1993; **90:** 1513–7.

51. Sellke FW, Wang SY, Friedman M et al. Basic FGF enhances endothelium-dependent relaxation of the collateral-perfused coronary microcirculation. *Am J Physiol* 1994; **267:** H1303–11.

52. Landau C, Jacobs AK, Haudenschild CC. Intrapericardial basic fibroblast growth factor induces myocardial angiogenesis in a rabbit model of chronic ischemia. *Am Heart J* 1995; **129:** 924–31.

53. Laham R, Rezaee M, Post M et al. A single intrapericardial dose of basic fibroblast growth factor induces functional angiogenesis in a porcine model of chronic myocardial ischemia. *Circulation* 1998; **98:** I-794 (abstr).

54. Watanabe E, Smith DM, Sun J et al. Effect of basic fibroblast growth factor on angiogenesis in the infarcted porcine heart. *Basic Res Cardiol* 1998; **93:** 30–7.

55. Uchida Y, Yanagisawa-Miwa A, Nakamura F et al. Angiogenic therapy of acute myocardial infarction by intrapericardial injection of basic fibroblast growth factor and heparan sulfate: an experimental study. *Am Heart J* 1995; **130:** 1182–8.

56. Horrigan M, MacIsaac A, Nicolini F et al. Reduction in myocardial infarct size by basic fibroblast growth factor after temporary coronary occlusion in a canine model. *Circulation* 1996; **94:** 1927–33.

57. Cuevas P, Carceller F, Ortega S et al. Hypotensive activity of fibroblast growth factor. *Science* 1991; **254:** 1208–10.

58. Cuevas P, Gonzalez AM, Carceller F, Baird A. Vascular response to basic fibroblast growth factor when infused onto the normal adventitia or into the injured media of the rat carotid artery. *Circ Res* 1991; **69:** 360–9.

59. Huang Z, Chen K, Huang P et al. bFGF ameliorates focal ischemic injury by blood flow-independent mechanism in eNOS mutant mice. *Am J Physiol* 1996; **272:** H1401–5.

60. Cuevas P, Carceller F, Lozano RM et al. Protection of rat myocardium by mitogenic and non-mitogenic fibroblast growth factor during post-ischemic reperfusion. *Growth Factors* 1997; **15:** 29–40.

61. Cuevas P, Reimers D, Carceller F et al. Fibroblast growth factor-1 prevents myocardial apoptosis triggered by ischemia reperfusion injury. *Eur J Med Res* 1972; **2:** 465–8.

62. Laham R, Sellke F, Edelman J, Simons M. Local perivascular basic fibroblast growth factor (bFGF) treatment in patients with ischemic heart disease. *J Am Coll Cardiol* 1998; **31:** 394A (abstr).

63. Laham R, Sellke F, Ware J et al. Results of a randomized, double-blind, placebo-controlled study of local perivascular basic fibroblast growth factor (bFGF) treatment in patients undergoing coronary artery bypass surgery. *J Am Coll Cardiol* 1999; (in press).

64. Laham R, Leimbach M, Chronos N et al. Intracoronary administration of recombinant fibroblast growth factor-2 (rFGF-2) in patients with severe coronary artery disease: results of phase I. *J Am Coll Cardiol* 1999; (in press).

# 15. The Intrapericardial Approach for Therapeutic Angiogenesis

Dongming Hou and Keith L March

## Introduction

Although percutaneous transluminal coronary angioplasty (PTCA) and bypass surgery are traditionally used in the prevention and treatment of ischemic heart disease, a large number of patients cannot tolerate these conventional methods owing to diffuse coronary artery disease, small vessels, or serious medical comorbidities. "Therapeutic angiogenesis" is a potential set of methods to enhance vascular growth to an area of ischemia. Angiogenesis, the formation of new vessels from pre-existing blood vessels, includes elements of sprouting and intussusceptive growth to form branches; and longitudinal vessel growth by intercalation of endothelial and other vascular cells. Intussusceptive growth forms capillary loops or subdivides a larger sinusoidal capillary into two smaller capillaries, while intercalation of endothelial cells increases the length and diameter of blood vessels.[1]

New vessels can improve myocardial perfusion and metabolism in ischemic regions. Numerous polypeptide growth factors and cytokines, both stimulators and inhibitors, influence angiogenesis. Angiogenic bioactive factors activate endothelial cells; angiogenic effect is thought to depend on the relative balance between positive and negative regulators to which the endothelial cell is exposed at any given time.[2,3]

## Therapeutic myocardial angiogenesis: approaches to delivery

The normal physiological response to tissue ischemia includes angiogenesis and recruitment of pre-existing collateral vessels in an effort to locally restore the required blood supply. However, the extent of this supplemented blood flow may not fully replace the normal flow in many cases. Optimal means to amplify the natural angiogenic response must be identified whenever possible. Numerous research groups have presented clear evidence of myocardial angiogenesis after local application of growth factors either in the ameroid constrictor animal model or in clinical trials. The goal of therapeutic angiogenesis is reduction of myocardium tissue hypoxia in ischemic areas. Most studies describing the application of angiogenic factors have employed: endovascular delivery via either intracoronary instillation or local intracoronary delivery devices, with single or multiple bolus doses of cytokine infusion; direct myocardial injection of vectors encoding angiogenic factors; epicardial placement of a polymeric or osmotic pump system to provide sustained delivery of desired agents; and direct intrapericardial space instillation. The studies have generally shown significant beneficial effects including enhanced myocardial neovascularization, improved coronary flow, reduced infarction size, and preserved regional haemodynamics.

Local delivery of a therapeutic agent to target disease regions while minimizing systemic toxic effects would seem to be a reasonable strategy for administration of highly potent agents, such as vascular growth factors, to the particular regions of need. It was hoped that local intracoronary delivery would allow the achievement of high concentrations of pharmacological drugs or therapeutic bioactive agents within the coronary artery wall. Although various endovascular delivery devices have been designed for this purpose, the limitations of such delivery include the possibility of increased vascular trauma, low efficiency of localization, inconsistency of delivery, and rapid washout of the agent from the vascular wall after delivery.[4,5] Several studies have shown that only 0.1 to 0.6% of agent remains in the artery wall after endovascular local delivery in porcine coronary vessels.[6] The inadequacy of intracoronary delivery may have recently been highlighted by the initial report of lack of efficacy in a phase II human trial involving bolus intracoronary injection of VEGF165 protein.[7] Accordingly, the alternative delivery approach of direct myocardial injection merits further exploration, which has been done most recently in studies of patients who received injection of aFGF protein[8,9] and naked plasmid DNA encoding phVEGF165 at the time of thoracotomy.[10] The initial results suggest that this approach is safe, and may lead to reduction of symptoms. Many aspects of the intramyocardial injection method remain under-developed, including the optimal dose and distribution of injection sites.

As an alternative to local intracoronary delivery or direct myocardial injection methods the pericardial space may be a suitable area for delivery of therapeutic angiogenic factors to the heart. The apparent benefits of delivering agents to the pericardial sac include: comparatively enhanced consistency of local agent levels; markedly reduced acute systemic delivery of agent; and prolonged exposure of either coronary or myocardial tissues to the therapeutic material as a result of a reservoir function of the pericardium. In experiments that compared endoluminal delivery with pericardial delivery of proteins including angiogenic growth factors, we have shown that contents instilled into the pericardial fluid can access coronary arteries with intramural concentrations that vary by 10–15 fold, while endoluminal delivery results in a notably wider intramural concentration range of up to 33 000-fold variability.[5] Figure 15.1 shows the

**190**

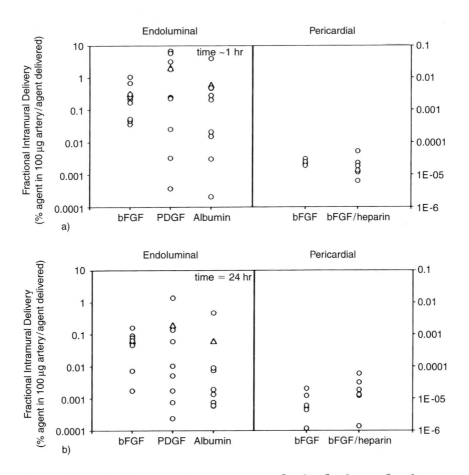

**Figure 15.1:** *(a) FID expressed as a percentage of each infused agent found in arterial tissue 1 h after delivery. The left panel shows one value for each coronary artery harvested after endoluminal delivery of the agents listed on the x-axis. The right panel shows one value for each coronary artery harvested following intrapericardial delivery of the indicated agents. It is apparent that endoluminal delivery results in greater degree of variation in FID by several orders of magnitude. (b) Fractional intramural retention (FIR) expressed as a percentage of each infused agent found in arterial tissue 24 h after delivery. The left panel shows one value for each coronary artery harvested after endoluminal delivery of the agents listed on the x-axis. The right panel shows one value for each coronary artery harvested following intrapericardial delivery of the indicated agents. It is apparent that endoluminal delivery results in a substantially greater degree of variation in FIR. bFGF = basic fibroblast growth factor, PDGF = platelet-derived growth factor. (From: Stoll HP et al. Pharmacokinetics and consistency of pericardial delivery directed to coronary arteries: direct comparison with endoluminal delivery.* Clin Cardiol *1999; 22 (suppl I): I-10–16, with permission.)*

**191**

fractional intramural delivery (FID) after endoluminal and pericardial deliveries, and indicates that the intrapericardial approach has a substantially greater reproducibility of localization.

## The pericardial space: ideal for delivery

The pericardium is a double-walled fibro-serous sac that encloses the heart and the roots of the great vessels. The potential space between the parietal and visceral layers of serous pericardium is called the pericardial space. It normally contains a small amount of clear fluid in human beings. Emerging data progressively suggest that the normal function of pericardial fluid is not only to prevent friction from occurring when the heart beats, but perhaps also to provide for a particular biochemical microenvironment that bathes the epicardial coronary vessels and myocardium. Recent studies have suggested that specific modulation of a number of angiogenic cytokines and growth factors occurs in the pericardial fluid in particular coronary disease conditions. According to one group, the concentration of bFGF (2036 $\pm$ 357 pg/ml $vs$ 289 $\pm$ 72 pg/ml, $p < 0.001$) and VEGF (39 $\pm$ 7 pg/ml $vs$ 22 $\pm$ 6 pg/ml, $p$ = NS) in the pericardial fluid of patients with unstable angina may be higher than in patients with non-ischemic heart disease.[11] Particular populations of patients have also shown variable content of angiogenic factors. [12,13] Changes in the cellular and molecular composition of pericardial fluid may reflect pathophysiological processes of myocardial ischemia and injury, as well as activation of macrophages and endothelial cells in the coronary vasculature.[14,15] Therefore, we hypothesized that the intrapericardial space may be a significant therapeutic site, because it is a "convenient" space with which to work; and also because there seems to be a natural process of growth factor exchange from the myocardium and its vessels into the pericardium and in the opposite direction.

## Intrapericardial delivery methods

Intrapericardial delivery has been done by several methods, including: pericardial sac exposure by thoracotomy followed by pericardial sac puncture; percutaneous transatrial and transventricular access; and percutaneous transthoracic approaches.

Lazarous and colleagues[16] used a 6.6F silastic catheter with end hole positioned into the pericardial space in dogs after a left thoracotomy. Differential regional uptake of [125]I-labeled bFGF was assessed in that study.

Recent technical advances have made available practical percutaneous methods for accessing the pericardial space. Transatrial access has been successfully used by Uchida and colleagues[17] and Verrier and colleagues[18]. Uchida and colleagues[17] used a thin needle-tipped catheter to deliver bFGF and heparin through the right atrium into the pericardial cavity in a canine model of acute myocardial infarction. Verrier and colleagues established a consistently successful transatrial approach for delivery. In their initial report, 19 animals (six dogs, 13 pigs) were tested using right or left femoral vein access to position a 6F or 8F-guide catheter in the right atrial appendage. A small perforation was made with a 21-gauge hollow radio-opaque needle catheter. This catheter was subsequently exchanged over a guidewire for a tapered-tip 4F-aspiration catheter with withdrawal side ports, permitting pericardial delivery and withdrawal of fluid. This study concluded that the transatrial approach provides a rapid means to access the pericardial space for delivery of therapeutic agents.

The transventricular method, demonstrated for adenoviral delivery[19] and more recently by Stoll and colleagues[20] for bFGF intrapericardial space instillation, uses a hollow, helical-tipped catheter designed for controlled penetration through the myocardium into the pericardial sac under fluoroscopic guidance. In this method, a catheter is placed through a right jugular or carotid sheath and advanced respectively into either the right or left ventricle to the cardiac free wall. On firm contact with the myocardium, the catheter tip is advanced through the myocardium with a gentle turning motion. After initial advancement, hand infusion of a 1:1 meglumine/normal saline mixture is begun and contrast location is monitored by fluoroscopy. Successful intrapericardial tip placement is shown by accumulation of contrast in the pericardium, and may be followed by delivery and device removal by rotation. The helical exit appears to preclude significant local bleeding. Figure 15.2 shows intrapericardial contrast delivery via a hollow helical-tipped catheter.

A percutaneous transthoracic delivery approach has been used by both Landau and colleagues[21] and Laham and colleagues.[22] Landau used transthoracic access to achieve intrapericardial bFGF delivery in a rabbit model. After partial surgical dissection to create a tunnel, a 22-gauge spinal needle assembly was directed at a 15-degree angle to the skin surface of the subxiphoid region and, using fluoroscopy, advanced left of midline towards the cardiac silhouette and through the diaphragm into the pericardial space. A guidewire and 5F dilator were then serially inserted, and after dilating the puncture tunnel, a 20 cm length of polyethylene tubing was advanced over the wire to the pericardial space. This tubing was connected with an osmotic pump for loading bFGF. Laham and colleagues used a blunt-tipped needle percutaneous subxiphoid access of the pericardial space procedure in the Yorkshire pig. In that study, animals underwent nonsurgical pericardial space bFGF or saline delivery 3 weeks after ameroid placement on the left circumflex artery.

Recently, a new pericardial access device called the PerDUCER® has been designed to minimize the possibility of myocardial puncture by the access needle

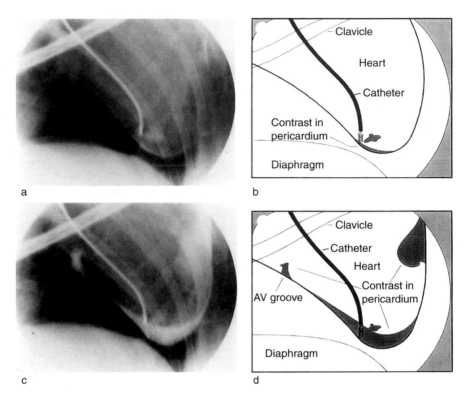

**Figure 15.2:** *Sequential fluorographic images, obtained during a percutaneous delivery procedure, from the right anterior oblique projection. (a) Cardiac silhouette, with the helix catheter in place transmurally in the right ventricular wall. The instillation of contrast had just begun at the time of angiography; a thin layer of contrast is seen outlining the cardiac edge, confirming pericardial location. This image is represented as a line drawing in (b) for clarity. (c) The same projection after the infusion of approximately 15 $cm^3$ of a mixture of radiographic contrast and vector suspension, with a line representation in (d). (From: March KL et al. Efficient in vivo catheter-based pericardial gene transfer mediated by adenoviral vectors.* Clin Cardiol *1999; 22 (suppl I): I-23–9, with permission.)*

during transthoracic access of a non-effused pericardial sac. This device is a needle protectively sheathed with a catheter bearing a hemispherical-shaped side-hole at its tip, which allows for the suction capture and subsequent puncture of the pericardium. Before using a PerDUCER®, a percutaneous tunnel is made below the xiphoid process using a 21-gauge needle introduced nearly parallel to the skin surface, after which an 0.038 inch diameter guidewire and introducer

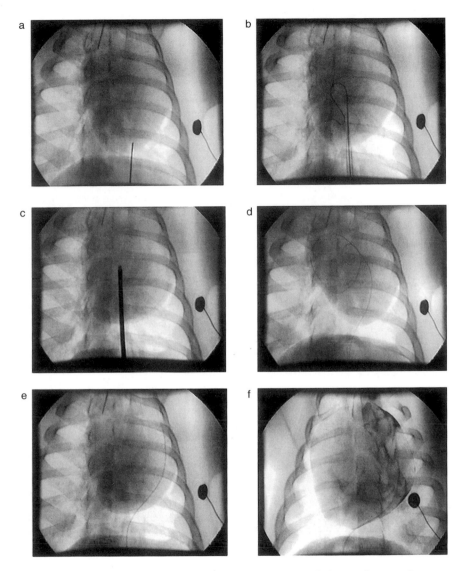

**Figure 15.3:** *Sequential fluorographic images, obtained during the procedure using PerDUCER®. (a) A percutaneous tunnel is made below the xiphoid process using a 21-gauge needle. (b) The 0.038-inch guidewire and special introducer sheath is placed into the mediastinum over the anterior pericardium. (c) The PerDUCER® is inserted via the sheath. (d) An 0.018-inch guidewire is placed through the PerDUCER®. (e) A 4F dilator catheter is entered into the pericardial space. (f) 5 ml of a mixture of contrast was injected into the sac.*

**195**

sheath is placed under fluoroscopic guidance into the mediastinum over the anterior pericardium. The PerDUCER® is positioned through the sheath onto the anterior (outer) surface of the pericardial sac, which is then drawn into the hemispherical-shaped tip by manual suction, and pierced by the needle. Finally, an 0.018 inch guidewire is placed through the needle lumen and advanced several cm to confirm its confinement within the pericardial space. The needle is removed and a 4F dilator catheter inserted over the wire. Successful intrapericardial tip placement is tested by injection of contrast into the pericardial space. Figure 15.3 shows intrapericardial delivery of contrast in this manner. Initial animal and clinical trials indicate that this procedure is a safe and effective method for percutaneous insertion of a guidewire into the normal pericardial space.[23]

## Efficacy of experimental intrapericardial delivery of angiogenesis agents

Table 15.1 provides a summary of the studies that have investigated intrapericardial placement of angiogenic agents. All studies cited demonstrate that the pericardial space is an efficacious, consistent, relatively rapid, and minimally invasive administration route for angiogenesis peptides.

To investigate the pharmacokinetics of bFGF after intrapericardial delivery, Lazarous and colleagues injected about 100 µg/kg [125]I-labeled bFGF into the pericardial space in dogs, and assessed disposition after 150 min. Pericardial

### Table 15.1 Intrapericardial delivery methods of the angiogenic factor bFGF

| Research groups | Approaches | Model | Publication date |
|---|---|---|---|
| Landau et al. | Transthoracic access implanted pump | Rabbit chronic ischemic model | 1995 |
| Uchida et al. | Transatrial access | Dog acute myocardial infarction model | 1995 |
| Lazarous et al. | Thoracotomy access | Normal dog | 1997 |
| Stoll et al. | Transventricular access | Normal pig | 1998 |
| Laham et al. | Transthoracic access | Pig chronic ischemic mode | 1998 |

administration gave enhanced cardiac bFGF delivery in comparison with the intracoronary and intravenous routes. 19% of the injected dose bFGF was present at 150 min after intrapericardial delivery, with labeled bFGF recovered over the entire epimyocardial surface. A transmural gradient of bFGF from epicardium to endocardium was described but not quantified. Our laboratory has recently developed a mathematical model for myocardial penetration and local pharmacokinetics of bFGF after a single intrapericardial delivery, and we tested this model after porcine deliveries.[20] Two doses of bFGF (30 µg, 200 µg) admixed with either [131]I- or [125]I-bFGF were delivered. Washout was assessed over 24 h by serial scintigraphy or by direct activity measurement to define agent loss from the region of interest. Epi-to-endocardial concentration gradients were established at 1 h and 24 h by gamma-counting of cylinders of myocardial tissue sectioned tangentially to the surface, at 300 micron step intervals. After intrapericardial delivery, epicardial bFGF concentrations were 164 ± 59 (mean ± SEM)-fold and endocardial concentrations were 15 ± 9-fold higher than serum concentrations. Similar gradients were maintained for 24 h after intrapericardial delivery, and the $T_{1/2}$ of bFGF in pericardial fluid was 21 h. These data support the concept that the pericardial space offers a kinetically advantageous administration route for angiogenic peptides, and suggest the possible efficacy of pericardial growth factor delivery for myocardial angiogenesis.

To examine whether angiogenesis and myocardial salvage occur in a canine model of acute myocardial infarction, Uchida and colleagues delivered 30 µg bFGF and 3 mg heparin sulfate into the pericardial space. The infarct weight/left ventricle weight after 1 month was decreased from 24 ± 5.2% and 25 ± 4.0% in groups receiving saline and heparin, to 18 ± 2.4% in bFGF alone, and 10 ± 1.8% bFGF plus heparin groups, respectively. The vascular density in the infarcted area of the outer layer was the largest in the bFGF plus heparin group; this vascular number was particularly larger in the subepicardial infarcted areas. This result indicated that intrapericardial bFGF, especially in conjunction with heparin, increases subepicardial angiogenesis and promotes myocardial salvage.

Landau and colleagues and Laham and colleagues reported the effects of intrapericardial bFGF delivery in two models of chronic myocardial ischemia. The first study tested a rabbit model of myocardial ischemia due to angiotensin II (AII)-induced left ventricular hypertrophy, with bFGF infused into the pericardial space by an osmotic pump. After 4 weeks, a highly localized angiogenic effect of bFGF was observed, with mean angiogenesis scores significantly higher in treated animals than in control groups. Laham and colleagues undertook similar studies using an ameroid constrictor on the left circumflex coronary artery of Yorkshire pigs, with intrapericardial single dose administration of bFGF (30 µg, 2 mg) or saline 3 weeks later. The bFGF groups had significant improvement in left circumflex artery resistance and endothelium-dependent vasodilation[22] as well as

**197**

in myocardial perfusion and regional function,[24] reflecting increased collateralization. These data further support the likelihood that intrapericardial delivery may be a helpful therapeutic strategy for the biochemical treatment of myocardial ischemia.

## Conclusion

Because some patients cannot be treated with PTCA or bypass surgery for ischemic heart disease, other methods must be explored. Increased angiogenesis may be a key to enhance successful recovery. Exploration of pericardial administration of angiogenic factors has been stimulated by three recent conceptual advances: recognition of the important part that the pericardial space may play in endogenous pathophysiology and modulation of ischemic heart events; evidence of the pharmacokinetic and localization advantages of intrapericardial space delivery; and the development of practical approaches for non-surgical access to the normal pericardium. Numerous pre-clinical experimental results have shown increases in vascular collateralization and promotion of myocardial salvage using intrapericardial strategies. It may thus be concluded that manipulation of the composition of intrapericardial fluid by administration of angiogenic factors such as bFGF, aFGF, and VEGF may provide an especially efficacious and consistent minimally-invasive method for increasing neoangiogenesis.

## Acknowledgment

The authors thank Teresa Knight for her excellent editorial assistance.

## References

1.  Karen SM, Judah F. Angiogenesis in cardiovascular disease. In: *Molecular Basis of Cardiovascular Disease*, 2nd edn. Kenneth RC (ed.). WB Saunders: Philadelphia 1999: 393–409.

2.  Pepper MS. Manipulating angiogenesis: from basic science to the bedside. *Arterioscler Thromb Vasc Biol* 1997; **17:** 605–19.

3.  Iruela-Arispe ML, Dvorak HF. Angiogenesis: a dynamic balance of stimulators and inhibitors. *Thromb Haemost* 1997; **78:** 672–7.

4.  March KL. Method of local gene delivery to vascular tissue. *Semin Intervent Cardiol* 1996; **1:** 215–23.

**198**

5.  Stoll HP, Carlson K, Keefer LK et al. Pharmacokinetics and consistency of pericardial delivery directed to coronary arteries: direct comparison with endoluminal delivery. *Clin Cardiol* 1999; **22** (suppl I): I-10–16.

6.  Lincoff AM, Weinberger J. Local drug delivery and endovascular radiation. In: *Comprehensive Cardiovascular Medicine*, 1st edn. Topol EJ (ed.). Lippincott-Raven: Philadelphia, 1998: 2433–52.

7.  Henry TD, Annex BH, Azin MA et al. Double blind, placebo controlled trial of recombinant human vascular endothelial growth factor- the VIVA trial. *J Am Coll Cardiol* 1999; **33**: 384A.

8.  Schumacher B, Stegmann T, Pecher P. The stimulation of neoangiogenesis in the ischemic human heart by the growth factor FGF: first clinical results. *J Cardiovasc Surg (Torino)* 1998; **39**: 783–9.

9.  Schumacher B, Pecher P, von Specht BU, Stegmann T. Induction of neoangiogenesis in ischemic myocardium by human growth factors: first clinical results of a new treatment of coronary heart disease. *Circulation* 1998; **24**: 645–50.

10. Losordo DW, Vale PR, Symes JF et al. Gene therapy for myocardial angiogenesis. *Circulation* 1998; **98**: 2800–4.

11. Fujita M, Ikemoto M, Kishishita M et al. Elevated basic fibroblast growth factor in pericardial fluid of patients with unstable angina. *Circulation* 1996; **94**: 610–3.

12. Dickson TJ, Gurudutt V, Nguyen AQ et al. Establishment of a clinically correlated human pericardial fluid bank: evaluation of intrapericardial diagnostic potential. *Clin Cardiol* 1999; **22** (suppl I): I-40–2.

13. Gurudutt VV, Nguyen AT, Kumfer KT et al. Growth factor components in human pericardial fluid: diminished angiogenic potential in aged and female populations. *J Am Coll Cardiol* 1999; **33**: 515A.

14. Gibson AT, Segal MB. A study of the composition of pericardial fluid with special reference to the probable mechanisms of fluid formation. *J Physiol* 1978; **277**: 367–77.

15. Corda S, Mebazza A, Gandolfini MP et al. Trophic effect of human pericardial fluid on adult cardiac myocytes. *Circ Res* 1997; **81**: 679–87.

16. Lazarous DF, Shou M, Stiber JA, et al. Pharmacodynamic of basic fibroblast growth factor: route of administration myocardial and systemic distribution. *Cardiovascular Research* 1997; **36**: 78–85.

17. Uchida Y, Yanagisawa-Miwa A, Fumitake N et al. Angiogenic therapy of acute myocardial infarction by intrapericardial injection of basic fibroblast growth factor and heparin sulfate. *Am Heart J* 1995; **130**: 1182–8.

18. Verrier RL, Waxman S, Lovett EG, Moreno R. Transatrial access to the normal pericardial space: a novel approach for diagnostic sampling, pericardiocentesis, and therapeutic interventions. *Circulation* 1998; **98**: 2331–3.

**199**

19. Woody M, Mehdi K, Zipes DP et al. High efficiency adenovirus-mediated pericardial gene transfer in vivo. *J Am Coll Cardiol* 1996; **27:** 31A.

20. Stoll HP, Szabo A, March KL. Sustained transmyocardial loading with bFGF following single intrapericardial delivery: local kinetics and tissue penetration. *Circulation* 1998; **98:** I-399.

21. Landau C, Jacobs AK, Haudenschild CC. Intrapericardial basic fibroblast growth factor induces myocardial angiogenesis in a rabbit model of chronic ischemia. *Am Heart J* 1995; **129:** 924–31.

22. Laham RJ, Simons M, Tofukuji M et al. Modulation of myocardial perfusion and vascular reactivity by pericardial basic fibroblast growth factor: insight into ischemia-induced reduction in endothelium-dependent vasodilatation. *J Thorac Cardiovasc Surg* 1998; **116:** 1022–8.

23. Seferovic PM, Ristic AD, Marsimovic R et al. Initial clinical experience with PerDUCER® device: promising new tool in the diagnosis and treatment of pericardial disease. *Clin Cardiol* 1999; **22** (suppl I): I-30–5.

24. Laham RJ, Sellke FW, Ware JA et al. Results of a randomized, double-blind, placebo-controlled study of local perivascular basic fibroblast growth factor (bFGF) treatment in patients undergoing coronary artery bypass surgery. *J Am Coll Cardiol* 1999; **33:** 383A.

# 16. Intramyocardial Injection of Acidic Fibroblast Growth Factor: Adjunct to Bypass Surgery and Monotherapy for Coronary Heart Disease

Thomas J Stegmann

## Summary

Currently available approaches for treating human coronary heart disease aim to relieve symptoms and the risk of myocardial infarction either by reducing myocardial oxygen demand, preventing further disease progression, restoring coronary blood flow pharmacologically or mechanically, or bypassing the stenotic lesions and obstructed coronary artery segments. Gene therapy, especially using angiogenic growth factors, has emerged recently as a potential new treatment for cardiovascular disease. After extensive experimental research on angiogenic growth factors, the first clinical studies on patients with coronary heart disease and peripheral vascular lesions have been done. The polypeptides fibroblast growth factor (FGF) and vascular endothelial growth factor (VEGF) appear to be particularly effective in initiating neovascularization (neoangiogenesis) in hypoxic or ischemic tissues. The first clinical study on patients with coronary heart disease treated by local intramyocardial injection of FGF1 showed a 3-fold increase of capillary density mediated by the growth factor. Angiogenic therapy of the human myocardium introduces a new method of treatment for coronary heart disease in terms of regulation of blood vessel growth. Beyond drug therapy, angioplasty, and bypass surgery, this new approach may become a fourth principle of treatment for atherosclerotic cardiovascular disease, especially for patients with diffuse disease not amenable to bypass surgery or PTCA, as well as adjunct to bypass surgery.

## Introduction

Whereas the role of angiogenesis in cancer and blood vessel development is well documented,[1] until now the use of angiogenesis to restore blood flow to ischemic tissue, especially the ischemic myocardium, has received less attention. Today, clinical applications of angiogenesis research focus on three general topics: antiangiogenic therapy (especially for tumors); prognostic markers in cancer patients; and angiogenic therapy (especially for ischemic tissues). The first attempt at angiogenic therapy for human ischemic peripheral vascular disease was the application of intra-arterial and intramuscular gene transfer of naked plasmid DNA encoding human VEGF in patients with severe vascular disease in the lower limbs.[2,3] The report of the worldwide first angiogenic therapy of coronary heart disease in humans was published by our group in 1994 and 1998.[4-6]

In established blood vessels in mature organisms, the endothelial cells remain in a quiescent, non-proliferative state until stimulation of angiogenesis occurs via conditions such as wounding, inflammation, hypoxia, or ischemia. The formation of new vessels is the result of several processes: dissolution of the matrix underlying the endothelial cell line; migration, adhesion, and proliferation of endothelial cells; formation of a new three-dimensional tube, which then lengthens from its tip as circulation is reestablished; for larger vessels, vascular smooth muscle cells migrate as well, and also adhere to the newly deposited matrix of the nascent vessel.[7] Angiogenic growth factors induce, promote, or interfere with all these steps of angiogenesis. In addition to their role in the initial development of the vascular system, angiogenic growth factors, like FGF and VEGF, and their receptors are expressed by endothelial cells in capillaries sprouting from established vessels in response to pathological conditions. Expression of receptors for FGF and VEGF varies according to the vascular bed, with little or no expression present in the normal myocardium, and can be altered by ischemia.[7] Reduction of oxygen tension promotes enhanced expression of mitogens, including FGF, VEGF, PDGF, and their receptors,[7] as well as endothelial cell growth.[8]

In particular, the heparin-binding growth factors – and FGF, VEGF are included in this group – have been tested in the treatment of experimental myocardial ischemia. In one of the first studies,[9] two intracoronary injections of FGF2 (basic) were given immediately following induction of acute myocardial infarction in dogs. Examination of the hearts 2 weeks later showed a reduction in the infarct size, as well as an increase in the number of capillaries and arterioles in the FGF2-treated animals. Another study with intracoronary injection of FGF2 in pigs with acute myocardial infarction also showed increased neovascularization in the treated animals, but failed to show any effect on left ventricular function.[10]

Essential benefits have also been obtained in models of chronic myocardial ischemia treated by heparin-binding growth factors.[11-14] Unlike the studies in acute ischemia, in which the growth factor was delivered only by intracoronary injections, growth factors have been given to animals with chronic ischemia by use of several techniques that permit sustained delivery; both extravascular and intravascular approaches have been tested.[14-16] FGF1 and FGF2 have been

**202**

reported to induce angiogenesis in the chronically ischemic porcine myocardium sufficient to improve myocardial perfusion and contractility, reduce infarct size, and normalize endothelium-dependent vascular reactivity.[9,10,13] In addition, viral-mediated gene transfer has recently been investigated as a method of delivery of angiogenic growth factors in an animal model of chronic ischemia – FGF5 given by adenoviral-mediated gene transfer increased perfusion in the ischemic myocardium as well as increased numbers of capillaries in both normal and ischemic tissue areas.[11]

Experimental application of modified fibrin glue with FGF1 between the descending aorta and the myocardium of the left ventricle resulted in the start of site-directed formation of new blood vessel structures to the heart.[15,16] A more recent study in rats with myocardial ischemia followed by creation of transmural channels (similar to the principle of transmyocardial laser revascularization TMR) showed a significant angiogenic response, in terms of raised expression of the FGF, TGF, and VEGF.[17]

This chapter summarizes our experimental and clinical experiences with FGF1. We describe first the experimental results that form the basis for clinical application of FGF1 in human beings. In the second part, we present a survey of our latest available clinical data of FGF1 therapy for coronary heart disease in humans, and data from our current clinical trials.

## Experimental preclinical research

The technique of gene transfer into apathogenic strains of *Escherichia coli* was used for producing human FGF1, and is described in detail elsewhere.[4,15,16] In summary, FGF-c-DNA plasmids in a total of 40 *E coli* cultures were submitted to clonal growth. After isolation and characterization by BIO-RAD-assay, further purification was done by SDS-electrophoresis and high-performance liquid chromatography (HPLC). The biochemical structure of isolated FGF1 was proved by western blot analysis using FGF1 IgG antibodies. Following this production process we achieved a 97% purity of FGF1 by SDS-PAGE; the growth factor then was lyophilized and stored at $-32°C$ (Figure 16.1).

For exclusion of any *oncogenic* or tumor-stimulating effects of FGF1, we did stimulation tests on various human tumor-cell strains as well as animal experiments. Four human tumor types were investigated: pleomorphic cell sarcoma, hypernephroma, melanoma, and small cell carcinoma of the bronchus. After 24 h-stimulation of tumor cell cultures by different concentrations of FGF1 (10 ng, 100 ng, control group without FGF1) no increase in the rate of DNA-synthesis by means of $^3$H-thymidine assay was found in the FGF1-groups compared with the control group. Additionally, tumor growth and tumor grading in a total of 320 naked mice – four groups of 80 animals each, with the

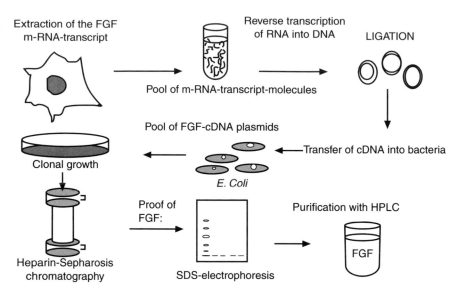

**Figure 16.1:** *Production of FGF1 by gene technology.*

four human tumor types (as indicated above) implanted ($3 \times 10^6$ cells) into the abdominal wall – were investigated and assessed 12 weeks after tumor-cell implantation. Tumor cells separately (40 animals), tumor cells and systemic FGF1 (40 animals), tumor cell/FGF1-suspension locally (40 animals), and FGF1 separately (40 animals) were applied. Measurements of the tumor sizes and weights following tumor explantation after 12 weeks showed no difference between the groups. There was also no difference in tumor grading by histological examination for all groups (Figure 16.2).

The question of *pyrogenic* effects of the purified growth factor FGF1 was evaluated in 40 white New Zealand rabbits (13 served as controls – injection of heat-denatured FGF1). Nine animals each received FGF1 (concentration: 0.01; 0.5; 1.0 mg/kg body weight) subcutaneously, intramuscularly, and intravenously. During the closely controlled follow-up period of 12 days there were no significant changes in rectal temperature, white cell count, erythrocyte sedimentation rate, and C-reactive protein values. These results, excluding pyrogenity of FGF1, were independent of the concentration of FGF1 and of its administration route (i.v., i.m., or s.c.).

The *angiogenic efficacy* of FGF1 was assessed in human venous endothelial cell cultures, in the chorio-allantoic membrane assay (CAM), and experimentally in 12 non-ischemic and 275 ischemic rat hearts (Lewis). Endothelial cell cultures were obtained from 40 segments of human great saphenous veins removed

**204**

| Tumor (80 nude mice/tumor) | Size of Tumor (cm) | | Grading (0-3) | |
|---|---|---|---|---|
| | with FGF1 | w/o FGF1 | with FGF1 | w/o FGF1 |
| Sarcoma | 2.6 | 2.8 | 3 | 3 |
| Hypernephroma | 1.2 | 1.1 | 1 | 1 |
| Melanoma | 0.8 | 0.9 | 2 | 3 |
| Bronchial-Ca. | 2.4 | 2.5 | 2 | 2 |

*Figure 16.2: Experimental research: histology of implanted human tumors in mice: 12-week results.*

during bypass surgery. From a total of 189 cell cultures with an initial cell density of $2.6 \times 10^4$ cells per $cm^2$, three groups were generated: group 1 (49 cultures) served as controls; to group 2 and to group 3 (70 cultures each) FGF1 was added in various concentrations: 0.02; 0.1; 0.2; 1.0; 2.0; 10.0; 20.0 ng FGF1 per ml cell suspension (10 cultures each); in group 3 additionally 1.0 mg heparin was enclosed. In all groups a confluent cell monolayer developed, in group 1 after 8 to 11 days, in group 2 (with FGF1) and in group 3 (with FGF1 plus heparin) after 5 to 8 days. By cell counting, a significant increase of cells was measured in groups 2 and 3 compared with the control group; additionally, for the FGF1 concentrations of 0.2 and 1.0 ng/ml the adjunct of heparin (group 3) resulted in a further increase of cell counts compared with group 2 (without heparin, $p < 0.01$). Also, the rate of DNA synthesis (tritiated thymidine counts, $cpm \times 10^3$; $^3H$-thymidine assay) showed a highly significant ($p < 0.005$) growth-promoting effect for human venous endothelial cells by FGF1 (group 2 and group 3) compared with the control cultures (group 1). And again, the adjunct of heparin (group 3) was followed by an additional increase of DNA-synthesis rate compared with the cultures without heparin (group 2), especially for the FGF1 concentrations 0.2, 1.0, and 2.0 ng/ml, respectively ($p < 0.01$).

In the CAM, 4 days after the application of FGF1 (10 ng) to the membrane (20 fertilized hen eggs, incubated for 13 days), the angiogenic effect of FGF1 could be shown under microscopy as radial growth of new vessels originating

**205**

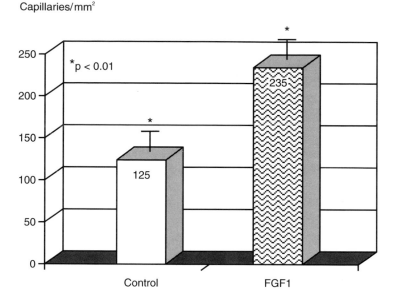

Capillaries/mm²

*Figure 16.3:* Experimental research: capillary density in ischemic rat hearts after 12 weeks.

from the original membrane vessels at the point of FGF1 application. New vasculature structures were completely absent in the control group (heat denatured FGF1). FGF1-induced neoangiogenesis was also shown in the non-ischemic rat heart: in 11 of 12 animals, 9 weeks after implantation of a FGF1/fibrin glue coated PTFE-membrane between the left ventricle and the descending thoracic aorta, a tissue with newly grown vascular structures could be observed on angiography, and confirmed histologically. In the control animals (n = 6, implantation of uncoated PTFE-membrane), no angiogenesis could be detected.

The induction of neoangiogenesis by FGF1 was then proved in the ischemic rat heart. A total of 275 Lewis rats was examined. After insertion of two titanium clips at the apex of the left ventricle, to create a myocardial ischemia in the distal part of the LAD area, 10 µg FGF1 was injected intramyocardially at the border region of the ischemic tissue (treated animals: n = 150). 125 animals not receiving FGF1 formed the control group. Aortic root angiography was done 12 weeks later in all surviving animals (88% in the FGF1 group, 82% in the control group). An increased accumulation of contrast medium was found in all treated animals in the region of the injected growth factor – in the borderline area between ischemic and normal myocardium. This accumulation was not

**206**

detectable in any of the control animals. Additionally, the histological examination of the myocardium where FGF1 was injected showed a significantly raised number of sectioned vessels, with an average of 235 capillaries per mm$^2$ in contrast to 125 capillaries per mm$^2$ in the control group (p <0.01, Figure 16.3). Furthermore, the numerous vessels seen in the myocardial sections of the treated animals revealed a normal three-layered vessel wall.

## Clinical results

After this extensive experimental testing of FGF1 in vitro and in vivo, our group undertook the world's first angiogenic therapy for human coronary artery disease in 1994–95, and we reported the results in 1994 and 1998.[4–6] In a randomized controlled clinical trial of 40 patients with three-vessel coronary artery disease who underwent bypass surgery, a simultaneous treatment by intramyocardial injection of FGF1 was accomplished in 20 patients. Twenty patients with intraoperative injection of heat-denatured FGF1 (70°C for 3 min) served as controls. All patients had a coronary pathology characterized – besides three-vessel-disease – by proximal LAD-stenosis with additional stenosis or occlusions of diagonal branches or the distal LAD. The ejection fraction of the left ventricle was greater than 40% in all patients. Both groups of patients had similar coronary pathology, clinical symptoms, cardiovascular risk factors, ventricular function, sex, age, and accompanying disorders. The choice of treatment was completely random, the names being placed in sealed envelopes and selected in a blinded manner. The study was approved and accepted by the Ethical Committee for Medical Research of the Phillips-University Marburg on August 10, 1993 (No. 47/93).

The operative bypass procedure was routinely done in all patients during extracorporal circulation with mild (30°C) hypothermia and cold cardioplegic arrest (St Thomas Hospital cardioplegic solution). All patients received an IMA bypass to the LAD, and additional venous grafts to the Cx and RCA system. The mean number of peripheral anastomosis for all 40 patients was 3.2. After completion of all distal anastomoses, and maintaining extracorporeal circulation, FGF1 (0.01 mg FGF1 per kg bodyweight) was intramyocardially injected distally to the IMA/LAD-anastomosis, close to the LAD and in direction to the additional peripheral stenosis/occlusion (diagonal branches, peripheral LAD). The growth factor solution was enriched by 1 ml fibrin glue and 1 mg heparin (Figure 16.4).

Twelve weeks (± 1) postoperatively in all patients the IMA-bypasses were imaged selectively by standardized transfemoral digital subtraction angiography, and recorded at a rate of four images per s. All angiograms were assessed by means of computer-assisted digital gray value analysis to show capillary

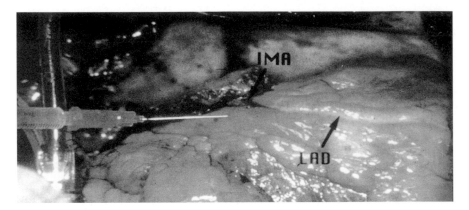

**Figure 16.4:** *Intraoperative intramyocardial injection of FGF1 into the human heart.*

neoangiogenesis in the areas of interest (ie, sites of intramyocardial injection of FGF1, or heat denatured FGF1, respectively).[4,5] All patients were followed up regularly until 3 years after angiogenic treatment by FGF1. As a result of the induction of myocardial neoangiogenesis by FGF1, a dense capillary network could be seen angiographically at the site of growth factor injection in all treated patients. This de novo vascular system enabled retrograde perfusion of stenosed diagonal branches as well as distally occluded segments of the LAD (Figure 16.5). In 20 control patients undergoing similar coronary bypass surgery in whom inactivated FGF1 was injected, there was no evidence of myocardial neovascularization on angiography at 12 weeks. The computer-assisted digital gray value analysis for quantification of neoangiogenesis confirmed a nearly 3-fold increase in myocardial vascularization for the FGF1 treated group compared with controls (gray value score 59 for the FGF1 group, 20 for the control group, p <0.005, Figure 16.6).

The follow-up results after 3 years (clinical examination, echocardiography, digital subtraction angiography of IMA-bypasses) also verified on the one side the prolonged and constant increase of vascularization at the FGF1-treated myocardial region, and on the other side the exclusion of any further or uncontrolled vessel growth (Figure 16.7). The gray value score amounted to a mean of 65 (3 months postoperatively: 59) in the FGF1-treated group compared with 18 (3 months postoperatively: 20) in the control group (bypass surgery plus heat denatured FGF1, p <0.005). Additionally, the results of the 3-year echocardiographic follow-up confirmed the angiographically demonstrated improvement of blood supply in the FGF1-treated group. The LV ejection fraction of the FGF1-treated group improved from 50.3% preoperatively to a

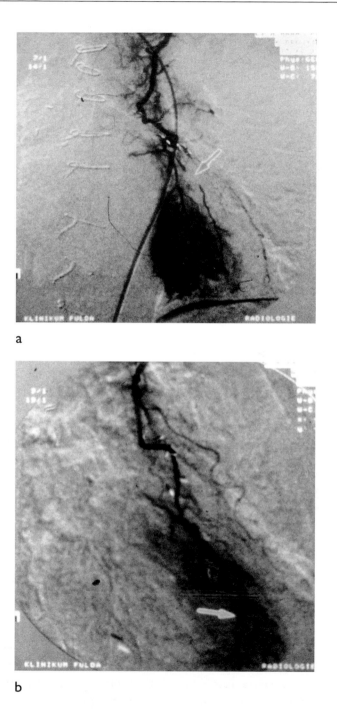

a

b

*Figure 16.5:* *Angiograms of patients 12 weeks after treatment by FGF1: newly grown arterial vessels are filling diagonal branches (a) or distal LAD (b). Arrows indicate occluded segments of a diagonal branch (a) and LAD (b).*

**209**

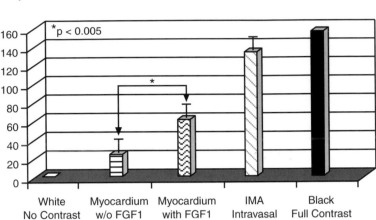

**Figure 16.6:** *Gray value analysis of FGF1 treated patients (= myocardium with FGF1) and control patients (= myocardium without FGF1).*

mean of 63.8% 3 years postoperatively. The corresponding values for the control group were 51.5% (preoperatively) and 59.4% (3 years postoperatively), respectively (Figure 16.8). Despite the fact that this was not a statistically significant difference, this finding showed some benefit for the patients treated simultaneously by bypass surgery and intramyocardial FGF1 application.

## Conclusions and outlook

In principal contrast to Isner and colleagues[2,3] our group[4-6] used FGF1 as angiogenic growth factor (not VEGF), employed directly the angiogenic growth factor (rather than gene transfer of plasmid DNA encoding the growth factor), and applied the angiogenic growth factor in close connection to the tissue area to be treated (in contrast to intra-arterial or intramuscular application). Thus, our procedure does not require the incorporation of DNA into the nucleus of the cells of the recipient tissue. We believe that our method therefore has the benefits of simplicity, predictability of dose, and circumscription of angiogenic growth factor effect. It seems of special interest in this context that with any kind of systemic application (or distribution) of the angiogenic growth factor some side effects may appear; in limited clinical experience plasmid-mediated VEGF gene therapy has led to development of exacerbation or initiation of local oedema, substantial systemic hypotension, or the risk of exacerbation of atherosclerotic plaque neovascularization resulting in plaque rupture.[18]

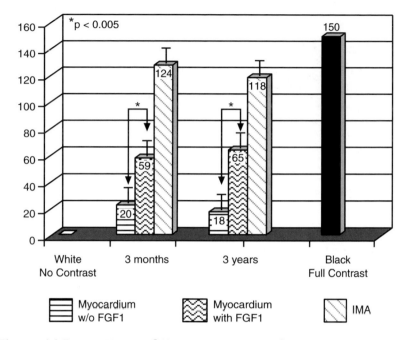

*Figure 16.7:* Late (3 years) follow-up: comparison of gray value analysis, 3 months versus 3 years.

All gene therapy designed to potentate local angiogenesis carries the theoretical risk that pathological angiogenesis at a remote site could be stimulated (eg, ocular angiogenesis or tumor angiogenesis).[1,19] Therefore, before considering the use of FGF1 in human patients, our group had to exclude any tumor-inducing or tumor-stimulating effects of FGF1 as well as in vitro assays as in numerous animal experiments of different species.[4-6] Also no pyrogenic side-effect of FGF1 was found. During our research neither an increase in the rate of growth of a tumor nor in its grading of malignancy followed the administration of FGF1. This may be most readily explained not only as a result of the specific binding of the factor to the high-affinity receptor system on the endothelial cell membrane, but also by the absence of hypoxia or ischemia as trigger for the activation of angiogenic potential of growth factors in other tissues.

Questions remain: is atherosclerotic plaque formation really angiogenesis (ie, FGF- and/or VEGF-) dependent? What is the optimal method to induce angiogenesis – application of plasmid DNA encoding VEGF or FGF, or direct

**211**

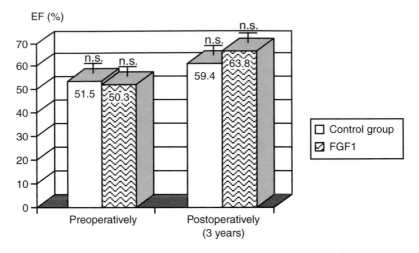

*Figure 16.8:* Late (3 years) follow-up: comparison of LV-ejection fraction (EF) between FGF1 group and control group of patients.

application of the angiogenic growth factor? Also the optimal route of administration, method of delivery, and toxic effects remain unresolved. And finally, questions of the best angiogenic growth factor or combination of growth factors in terms of angiogenic efficacy, singleness of directed angiogenesis, and minimized side-effects have to be answered. Further clinical studies on therapeutic induction of neoangiogenesis in patients with coronary heart disease must include well defined endpoints (ie, death, angina, exercise tolerance), angiographic endpoints (eg, quantification of new vessels or collaterals, assessment of coronary blood flow); and functional endpoints (ie, assessment of myocardial perfusion via perfusion scanning methods or NMR-techniques, and of global and regional left ventricular function at rest and exercise).

Following these guidelines, in 1998 our group started a second clinical trial to further investigate FGF1 efficacy as sole angiogenic therapy for patients with symptomatic coronary artery disease not amenable to bypass surgery or interventional techniques (Ethical Committee for Medical Research of the Phillips-University Marburg, No. 121/98). Via limited left anterior thoracotomy, FGF1 (0.01 mg/kg body weight) is injected into the target region of ischemic myocardium in accordance with the preoperative coronary angiogram. Follow-up includes control coronary angiography 12 weeks later, echocardiography during rest and exercise (stress-echocardiography), and SPECT perfusion scanning, respectively. Similar to Losordo and colleagues[20] our preliminary results in the first six patients (five men, one woman) of this study suggest: no operative mortality and morbidity; no significant changes in the hemodynamic status of the

**212**

patients; and clinical improvement of all six patients in terms of decrease or removal of angina.

Promotion of neovascularization in patients with ischemic cardiovascular disease has many attractive features; data available in preclinical and in the most recent clinical studies suggest that the induction of neoangiogenesis by angiogenic growth factors may provide revascularization in patients with ischemic heart disease for whom no alternative therapy currently exists. After the first promising results with angiogenic therapy of patients with coronary heart disease by local application of FGF1[4–6] our group suggests, that this new treatment method may become an additional option in the near future for those patients who have the *diffuse type* of coronary artery disease not amenable to established interventional procedures (like PTCA) or bypass surgery, and/or who have proximal coronary artery lesions (accessible for PTCA and/or bypass surgery) and *additional distal stenoses* or occlusions of the coronary vascular bed not accessible for PTCA and/or bypass surgery.[21] In these conditions, angiogenic therapy by intramyocardial injection of angiogenic growth factors like FGF1 could serve as an adjunct to routine bypass surgery for coronary heart disease.

# References

1.    Folkman J. Clinical applications of research on angiogenesis. *N Engl J Med* 1995; **333:** 1757–63.

2.    Isner JM, Pieczek A, Schainfeld R et al. Clinical evidence of angiogenesis after arterial gene transfer of ph $VEGF_{165}$ in patients with ischemic limb. *Lancet* 1996; **348:** 370–4.

3.    Baumgartner J, Pieczek A, Manor O et al. Constitutive expression of ph $VEGF_{165}$ after intramuscular gene transfer promotes collateral vessel development in patients with critical limb ischemia. *Circulation* 1998; **97:** 1114–23.

4.    Schlaudraff K, von Specht BU, Kolvenbach H et al. Induktion neuer funktioneller Blutgefäβe beim Menschen durch den ersten klinischen Einsatz des humanen Wachstumsfaktors HBGF-1. *Langenbeck Arch Chir Chirurg Forum* 1994; **54:** 167–72.

5.    Schumacher B, Pecher P, von Specht BU, Stegmann TJ. Induction of neoangiogenesis in ischemic myocardium by human growth factors. First clinical results of a new treatment of coronary heart disease. *Circulation* 1998; **97:** 645–50.

6.    Schumacher B, Stegmann TJ, Pecher P. The stimulation of neoangiogenesis in the ischemic human heart by the growth factor FGF: first clinical results. *J Cardiovasc Surg* 1998; **39:** 783–9.

7.    Ware JA, Simons M. Angiogenesis in ischemic heart disease. *Nature Med* 1997; **3:** 158–64.

8.      Kuwabara K, Ogawa S, Matsumoto M et al. Hypoxia-mediated induction of acidic/basic fibroblast growth factor and platelet-derived growth factor in mononuclear phagocytes stimulates growth of hypoxic endothelial cells. *Proc Natl Acad Sci USA* 1995; **92:** 4606–10.

9.      Yanagisawa-Miwa A, Uchida Y, Nakamura F et al. Salvage of infarcted myocardium by angiogenic action of basic fibroblast growth factor. *Science* 1992; **257:** 1401–3.

10      Battler A, Scheinowitz M, Bor A et al. Intracoronary injection of basic fibroblast growth factor enhances angiogenesis in infarcted swine myocardium. *J Am Coll Cardiol* 1993; **22:** 2001–6.

11.     Giordano FJ, Ping P, McKirnan MD et al. Intracoronary transfer of fibroblast growth factor-5 increases blood flow and contractile function in an ischemic region of the heart. *Nature Med* 1996; **2:** 534–9.

12.     Lazarous DF, Scheinowitz M, Shou M et al. Effects of chronic systemic administration of basic fibroblast growth factor on collateral development in the canine heart. *Circulation* 1995; **91:** 145–53.

13.     Harada K, Grossman W, Friedman M et al. Basic fibroblast growth factor improves myocardial function in chronically ischemic porcine hearts. *J Clin Invest* 1994; **94:** 623–30.

14.     Unger EF, Banai S, Shou M et al. Basic fibroblast growth factor enhances myocardial collateral flow in a canine model. *Am J Physiol* 1994; **266:** 1588–95.

15.     Fasol R, Schumacher B, Schlaudraff K et al. Experimental use of a modified fibrin-glue to induce site-directed angiogenesis from the aorta to the heart. *J Thorac Cardiovasc Surg* 1994; **107:** 1432–9.

16.     Schlaudraff K, Schumacher B, von Specht BU et al. Growth of new coronary vascular structures by angiogenetic growth factor. *Eur J Cardiothorac Surg* 1993; **7:** 637–44.

17.     Pelletier MP, Giaid A, Sivaraman S et al. Angiogenesis and growth factor expression in a model of transmyocardial revascularization. *Ann Thorac Surg* 1998; **66:** 12–18.

18.     Kuzuya M, Satake S, Esaki T et al. Induction of angiogenesis by smooth muscle cell-derived factor: possible role in neovascularization in atherosclerotic plaque. *J Cell Physiol* 1995; **164:** 658–67.

19.     Stegmann TJ. FGF1 a human growth factor in the induction of neoangiogenesis. *Exp Opin Invest Drugs* 1998; **7:** 2011–5.

20.     Losordo DW, Vale PR, Symes JF et al. Gene therapy for myocardial angiogenesis. *Circulation* 1998; **98:** 2800–4.

21.     Stegmann TJ. New approaches to coronary heart disease: induction of neovascularization by growth factors. *Bio Drugs* 1999; **11:** 301–8.

# 17. FIBROBLAST GROWTH FACTOR-1 (FGF1) GENE THERAPY FOR ISCHEMIC ARTERIAL DISEASE

Richard Pilsudski, Abder Mahfoudi, Bertrand Schwartz, Didier Branellec and Fabienne Soubrier

## Angiogenesis: generalities

The process of angiogenesis is orchestrated by a balance of angiogenic and angiostatic factors spatially and temporally regulated in vivo. It can be considered as the culmination of several steps, starting with exposure of a pre-existing vessel to an exogenous stimulus, degradation of the extracellular matrix underlying the endothelium, proliferation migration, and adhesion of endothelial cells, and, finally, organization into three-dimensional tubes (sprouting) that re-establishes blood supply to the ischemic area. In vessels larger than capillaries, vascular smooth muscle cells migrate as well, and adhere to the matrix deposited by the nascent vessel.

Manipulation of any of these factors might abolish, accelerate or induce angiogenesis. Since the pioneering work of Folkman[1] an extended literature has accumulated describing not only proangiogenic and antiangiogenic factors, but also the therapeutic potential for angiogenesis.[2]

## Therapeutic angiogenesis

The concept of using the angiogenic activity of a growth factor for a clinical application was first proposed by Folkman.[3] Therapeutic angiogenesis[4] is an approach that applies to the treatment of ischemia in a number of diseases such as limb ischemia, myocardial ischemia, and wound healing.

Acidic fibroblast growth factor (FGF1) is one of the first factors that was described to activate endothelial cell migration and proliferation in vitro.[5] FGF1 was also shown to induce angiogenesis in vivo when injected as a purified protein or when expressed from its DNA coding sequence inserted into an expresion vector.

# FGF1

FGFs are pleiotropic growth factors acting on endothelial cells, smooth muscle cells and fibroblasts via an interaction with specific receptors of the cell surface. Tissue distribution of FGF-receptors is wide, including brain, bone matrix, kidney, retina, heart, and many other tissues.

The gene encoding acidic fibroblast growth factor (FGF1), is one of the first factors that was shown to activate endothelial cell migration and proliferation in vitro. FGF1 was clearly shown to induce angiogenesis in vivo when injected as a purified protein or when expressed from its DNA coding sequence inserted in an expression vector.

## Recombinant protein

The first attempt to demonstrate the therapeutic potential of FGF1 was reported in 1991[6] in a dog model of chronic heart ischemia. In that study, interdisposition of sponge saturated with recombinant FGF1 between the internal mammary artery and ischemic myocardium did not induce bridging collateral formation. Interestingly, a mutant form of FGF1 with a longer activity half-life when compared to the wild type protein, was shown to have a significant activity on myocardial flow when formulated into ethylene vinyl acetate copolymer matrix and applied to the ameroid-compromised myocardium of pigs.[7] Pu and colleagues[8] studied the therapeutic effect of FGF1 in a rabbit model of hindlimb ischemia, and showed that daily intramuscular injection of recombinant FGF1 (4 mg) over 10 days could lead to a significant improvement of ischemic hindlimb deficit, based on angiographic and calf blood pressure assessments. Nabel and colleagues[9] also showed that recombinant FGF1 was able to promote intimal hyperplasia and angiogenesis in arteries in vivo.

The FGF1 protein was shown, in various experimental settings, to promote angiogenesis. These and other results prompted the initiation of clinical trials. Schumacher and colleagues[10] recently reported first clinical results of FGF1 recombinant protein (rFGF1) to induce neoangiogenesis in the ischemic myocardium of patients with coronary artery disease. rFGF1 was injected close to the vessels after the completion of internal mammary artery/left anterior descending coronary artery anastomosis in 20 patients with three vessel coronary disease. The formation of new capillaries was demonstrated in all cases around the site of injection. Angiography 12 weeks later showed coronary artery neovascularization extending out from the area of rFGF1 injection. Stenoses distal to the anastomosis were bridged by neovascularization. In 20 patients undergoing similar coronary artery bypass surgery in whom inactivated rFGF1 was injected, there was no evidence of myocardial neovascularization on 12-week angiography.

Very interestingly, FGF1, in addition to its proangiogenic properties, presents cardioprotective and anti-apoptotic effect in cardiac ischemia-reperfusion models; this was demonstrated both in pig[11] and rat models.[12] A similar effect might also be operative in skeletal muscle.[13]

## Gene therapy

Apart from recombinant protein injection, gene transfer provides a seductive alternative strategy to deliver locally sustained levels of protein. The feasibility of this approach was shown with FGF1 in a series of preclinical settings. Mühlhauser and colleagues[14] reported that subcutaneous administration of a replication deficient recombinant adenovirus expressing FGF1 fused to a heterologous secretion signal (from FGF4) resulted into angiogenesis in mice at the site of injection. Subsequently, Safi and colleagues[5] showed that intramyocardial injection of the FGF1 adenoviral vector before coronary artery ligation could induce angiogenesis in a rabbit model of myocardial infarction. Catheter-mediated transfer of a plasmid encoding a naturally occurring truncated form of human FGF1 fused to a heterologous secretion signal (sp.FGF1) was shown to promote angiogenesis in an animal model of experimental hindlimb ischemia.[15]

Gene therapy will require a careful selection of the vectors for each specific application. Basically, the choice is between viral vectors – the most advanced candidates being adenovirus and adeno-associated virus – and non-viral vectors.

Viral vectors can readily provide a high efficiency of gene transfer. This advantage has been shown clearly in the myocardium, comparing gene transfer after plasmid or adenoviral intramuscular injection.[16] Adeno-associated viruses also provide high levels of gene transfer, as demonstrated in peripheral and cardiac settings.[17,18] Viral vectors also offer the advantage of allowing for administration via infusion into the coronary artery, thus eliminating the need for open-chest surgery. Both routes of administration have been used to show that administration of adenoviral vectors encoding growth factors could provide a clinical improvement in porcine models of coronary artery diseases.[19]

The non-viral option is very seductive, being devoid of the viral-related drawbacks of immune response induction and inflammatory risks.[20] Moreover, as the gene transfer is very restricted to the injection site,[21] with no occurrence of integration described to date, this approach is judged particularly safe.[22]

Four clinical trials recently disclosed the safety and efficacy associated with this non-viral naked DNA injection process.[23–26] Striated muscle is capable of taking up and expressing genes from naked expression plasmids. Although direct intramuscular injection of plasmids is associated with moderate gene transfer, therapeutic efficacy (proangiogenic) was shown with genes encoding secreted angiogenic factors injected in the vicinity of arterial occlusion in animal models of

**217**

chronic limb ischemia[27–31] and in patients with severe peripheral artery disease,[25] Buerger's disease,[26] or ischemic heart disease.[32] This suggests that moderate gene expression may be compensated by a paracrine effect of angiogenic factors.

Efforts to improve eukaryotic expression plasmids for non-viral gene therapy have focused mainly on the improvement of transgene expression or plasmid copy number. However, none of the reported modifications, to our knowledge, attempted to integrate environmental, safety, and industrial requirements in the design of plasmid backbone.

We have also used the non-viral approach for the treatment of ischemic arterial disease using the FGF1 gene as a therapeutic gene. We developed very narrow-host range plasmids harboring an optimized FGF1 expression cassette inserted in a novel plasmid backbone design with conditional origin of replication (pCOR, Sourbrier and colleagues, unpublished data).

## Conclusions

Our data support the use of pCOR plasmid encoding FGF1 as a therapeutic tool for management of ischemic arterial disease. Based on these data, we will initiate two phase I clinical safety and biological activity studies to evaluate pCOR expressing FGF1. The first phase I will be done in patients with severe peripheral artery occlusive disease. Increasing single doses of pCOR expressing FGF1 will be administered into calf or distal thigh muscle of the ischemic limb. The second phase I study will be done in patients with refractory coronary artery disease who are poor candidates for angioplasty or bypass. pCOR plasmid expressing FGF1 will be injected into the myocardium via left ventricular endocardial delivery at selected sites in the ischemic area(s) and adjacent regions.

## References

1.   Folkman J. Tumor angiogenesis: therapeutic implications. *N Engl J Med* 1971; **285:** 1182–6.

2.   Van Belle E, Bauters C, Asahara T, Isner JM. Endothelial regrowth after arterial injury: from vascular repair to therapeutics. *Cardiovasc Res* 1998; **38:** 54–68.

3.   Folkman J. The angiogenic activity of FGF and its possible clinical applications. In: *Growth Factors: from Genes to Clinical Applications.* Sara VR et al (eds). Raven Press: New York, 1991: 201–16.

4.   Hockel M, Schlenger K, Doctrow S, Kissel T, Vaupel P. Therapeutic angiogenesis. *Arch Surg* 1993; **128:** 423–9.

5. Safi J, Gloe TR, Riccioni T, Kovesdi I, Capogrossi M. Gene therapy with angiogenic factors: a new potential approach to the treatment of ischemic disease. *J Mol Cell Cardiol* 1997; **29:** 2311–25.

6. Banai S, Jaklitsch MT, Casscells W et al. Effects of acidic fibroblast growth factor on normal and ischemic myocardium. *Circ Res* 1991; **69:** 76–85.

7. Lopez JJ, Edelman ER, Stamler A et al. Angiogenic potential of perivascularly delivered aFGF in a porcine model of chronic myocardial ischemia. *Am J Physiol* 1998; **274:** H930–6.

8. Pu LQ, Sniderman AD, Brassard R et al. Enhanced revascularization of the ischemic limb by angiogenic therapy. *Circulation* 1993; **88:** 208–15.

9. Nable EG, Yang ZY, Plautz G et al. Recombinant fibroblast growth factor-1 promotes intimal hyperplasia and angiogenesis in arteries in vivo. *Nature* 1993; **362:** 844 6.

10. Schumacher B, Pecher P, von Specht BU, Stegmann T. Induction of neoangiogenesis in ischemic myocardium by human growth factors. First clinical results of a new treatment of coronary heart disease. *Circulation* 1998; **97:** 645–50.

11. Htun P, Ito W, Hoefer I et al. Intramyocardial infusion of FGF1 mimics ischemic preconditioning in pig myocardium. *J Mol Cell Cardiol* 1998; **30:** 867–77.

12. Cuevas P, Carceller F, Hernandez-Madrid A et al. Protective effects of acidic fibroblast growth factor against cardiac arrhythmias induced by ischemia and reperfusion in rats. *Eur J Med Res* 1997; **2:** 33–46.

13. Fu X, Cuevas P, Gimenez-Gallego G et al. Acidic fibroblast growth factor reduces rat skeletal muscle damage caused by ischemia and reperfusion. *Chin Med J* 1995; **108:** 209–14.

14. Muhlhauser J, Pili R, Merrill MJ et al. In vivo angiogenesis induced by recombinant adenovirus vectors coding either for secreted or nonsecreted forms of acidic fibroblast growth factor. *Hum Gene Ther* 1995; **6:** 1457–65.

15. Tabata H, Silver M, Isner JM. Arterial gene transfer of acidic fibroblast growth factor for therapeutic angiogenesis in vivo: critical role of secretion signal in use of naked DNA. *Cardiovasc Res* 1997; **35:** 470–9.

16. Kass-Eisler A, Leinwand L. DNA and adenovirus-mediated gene transfer into cardiac muscle. *Methods Cell Biol* 1998; **52:** 423–37.

17. Kessler P, Podsakoff G, Chen X et al. Gene delivery to skeletal muscle results in sustained expression and systemic delivery of a therapeutic protein. *Proc Natl Acad Sci USA* 1996; **93:** 14082–7.

18. Fisher K, Jooss K, Alston J et al. Recombinant adeno-associated virus for muscle directed gene therapy. *Nat Med* 1997; **3:** 306–12.

19. Giordano F, Ping P, McKirnan M et al. Intracoronary gene transfer of fibroblast

growth factor-5 increases blood flow and contractile function in an ischemic region of the heart. *Nat Med* 1996; **2:** 534–9.

20. Gilgenkrantz H, Duboc D, Juillard V et al. Transient expression of genes transferred in vivo into heart using first generation adenoviral vectors: role of the immune response. *Hum Gene Ther* 1995; **6:** 1256–74.

21. Winegar R, Monforte J, Suing K et al. Determination of tissue distribution of an intramuscular plasmid vaccine using PCR and in situ DNA hybridization. *Hum Gene Ther* 1996; **7:** 2185–94.

22. Wolff J, Ludtke J, Acsadi G et al. Long-term persistence of plasmid DNA and foreign gene expression in mouse muscle. *Hum Mol Genet* 1992; **1:** 363–9.

23. MacGregor R, Boyer J, Ugen K et al. First human trial of a DNA-based vaccine for treatment of human immunodeficiency virus type 1 infection: safety and host response. *J Infect Dis* 1998; **178:** 92–100.

24. Wang R, Doolan D, Le T et al. Induction of antigen-specific cytotoxic T lymphocytes in humans by a malaria DNA vaccine. *Science* 1998; **282:** 476–80.

25. Baumgartner I, Pieczek A, Manor O et al. Constitutive expression of phVEGF165 after intramuscular gene transfer promotes collateral vessel development in patients with critical limb ischemia. *Circulation* 1998; **97:** 1114–23.

26. Isner JM, Baumgartner I, Rauh G et al. Treatment of thromboangiitis obliterans (Buerger's disease) by intramuscular gene transfer of vascular endothelial growth factor: preliminary clinical results. *J Vasc Surg* 1998; **28:** 964–73.

27. Takeshita S, Isshiki T, Mori H et al. Microangiographic assessment of collateral vessel formation following direct gene transfer of vascular endothelial growth factor in rats. *Cardiovasc Res 1997;* **35:** 547–52.

28. Tsurumi Y, Kearney M, Chen D et al. Treatment of acute limb ischemia by intramuscular injection of vascular endothelial growth factor gene. *Circulation* 1997; **96:** 382–8.

29. Takeshita S, Isshiki T, Ochiai M et al. Endothelium-dependent relaxation of collateral microvessels after intramuscular gene transfer of vascular endothelial growth factor in a rat model of hindlimb ischemia. *Circulation* 1998; **98:** 1261–3.

30. Shyu K, Manor O, Magner M et al. Direct intramuscular injection of plasmid DNA encoding angiopoietin-1 but not angiopoietin-2 augments revascularization in the rabbit ischemic hindlimb. *Circulation* 1998; **98:** 2081–7.

31. Witzenbichler B, Asahara T, Murohara T et al. Vascular endothelial growth factor-C (VEGF-C/VEGF-2) promotes angiogenesis in the setting of tissue ischemia. *Am J Pathol* 1998; **153:** 381–94.

32. Losordo D, Vale P, Symes J et al. Gene therapy for myocardial angiogenesis: initial clinical results with direct myocardial injection of phVEGF 165 as sole therapy for myocardial ischemia. *Circulation* 1998; **98:** 2800–4.

# 18. The Biosense™ Guided Transendocardial Injection System for Therapeutic Myocardial Angiogenesis

Ran Kornowski, Shmuel Fuchs, Stephen E Epstein and Martin B Leon

## Introduction

A novel approach that may have important application in the treatment of cardiovascular disease has been the use of recombinant genes or growth factors injected directly into the myocardium. Animal studies have proved the feasibility of introducing recombinant genes into cardiomyocytes by use of a direct intramyocardial injection approach.[1,2] The transfer of specific genes, controlled by suitable promotors, can cause the production of angiogenic proteins in ischemic areas.[3-6] The idea of this approach is to induce therapeutic angiogenesis through direct intramyocardial application of angiogenic proteins, or plasmids (naked DNA), or adenovirus-mediated gene transfer.[3-6] The effect of direct intraoperative intramyocardial injection of angiogenic factors on collateral function has been reported in experimental models, and angiogenesis is also being studied after direct intramyocardial injection of angiogenic peptides or plasmid vectors during open heart surgery in patients.[3-6] Catheter-based transendocardial injection of angiogenic factors may provide equivalent benefit without the need for surgery.

The Biosense™ system has been used for electromechanical mapping of the heart. This guidance system uses low-intensity magnetic field energy and sensor-tipped catheters to locate the catheter position in space, enabling a 3D image reconstruction of the left ventricle (LV), and enabling identification of ischemic target zones based on electromechanical endocardial signals to be obtained without x-ray exposure.[7,8] Once electroanatomical reconstruction of the LV is completed, the mapping catheter is removed from the LV and replaced by an 8F-tip injection catheter.

# The Biosense™ guided injection system

The Biosense injection catheter (Biosense \ Cordis-Webster, Johnson & Johnson, USA) is an investigational electromechanical mapping catheter modified to integrate a retrievable 27G nitinol needle for LV intramyocardial injection. The catheter "dead-space" is approximately 0.1 ml. The needle is controlled by a handle mechanism located proximal to the standard deflection handle (Figure 18.1). The injection handle has a Luer fitting for connection to a 1 or 3 cm$^3$ syringe (Figure 18.1). Standard operation of the syringe attached to the injection handle delivers the drug to the myocardium. The operator of the syringe controls the dosage using the graduations on the syringe. The exact catheter-tip location, orientation, and the injection sites are indicated in real-time on the LV

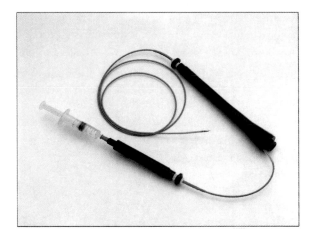

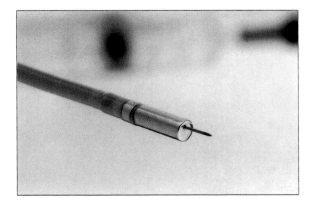

*Figure 18.1: The Biosense injection catheter integrates the mapping catheter with a retrievable 27G nitinol needle for LV transendocardial injection. The needle is controlled by a handle mechanism located proximal to the standard deflection handle. The injection handle has a Luer fitting for connection to a 1 or 3 cm$^3$ syringe. The 8F distal end of the injection catheter is equipped with a tip and ring electrodes, a location sensor, and a 27G nitinol needle designed for transendocardial injection.*

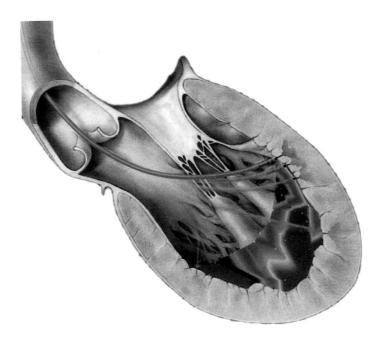

**Figure 18.2:** *Composite illustrated picture to show the ability of the Biosense transendocardial injection catheter to map the LV endocardial surface, to identify ischemic target regions (based on color-coded electromechanical signals) and to access designated regions of the left ventricle for gene delivery.*

electroanatomical map, and local electrical and location signals are traced to assure catheter stability and optimal endocardial contact (Figure 18.2).

We have recently shown that such a percutaneous magnetic-field guided approach for intramyocardial injection allows delivery of gene products into prespecified treatment zones. This has been achieved despite endocardial motion, and without perforation or other undesirable tissue effects or serious ventricular arrhythmias.[9,10] Moreover, a comparison of the transendocardial to transepicardial modes of administration, by use of β-galactosidase as a marker gene, showed no difference in the frequency or size of regions positive for β-galactosidase between the two gene-delivery approaches.

Thus, by use of this magnetic guided system, this investigational catheter-based intramyocardial gene-delivery system may be used in the future to treat the ischemic myocardium with angiogenic genes, proteins, or both, to enhance myocardial perfusion and function in a wide variety of patients with ischemic coronary syndrome.

## Acknowledgement

We gratefully acknowledge Richard A Gersony MFA, for his medical illustrations.

## References

1. Guzman RJ, Lemarchand P, Crystal RG et al. Efficient gene transfer into myocardium by direct injection of adenovirus vectors. *Circ Res* 1993; **73:** 1202–7.

2. Svensson EC, Marshall DJ, Woodard K et al. Efficient and stable transduction of cardiomyocytes after intramyocardial injection or intracoronary perfusion with recombinant adeno-associated virus vectors. *Circulation* 1999; **99:** 201–5.

3. Mack CA, Patel SR, Schwartz EA et al. Biologic bypass with the use of adenovirus-mediated gene transfer of the complementary deoxyribonucleic acid for VEGF-12, improves myocardial perfusion and function in the ischemic porcine heart. *J Thorac Cardiovasc Surg* 1998; **115:** 168–77.

4. Schumacher B, Peher P, von Specht BU, Stegman T. Induction of neoangiogenesis in ischemic myocardium by human growth factors. First clinical results of a new treatment of coronary heart disease. *Circulation* 1998; **97:** 645–50.

5. Losordo DW, Vale PR, Symes JF et al. Gene therapy for myocardial angiogenesis: initial clinical results with direct myocardial injection of phVEGF165 as sole therapy for myocardial ischemia. *Circulation* 1998: **98:** 2800–4.

6. Rosengart TK, Patel SR, Lee LY et al. Safety of direct myocardial VEGF-121 cDNA adenovirus-mediated angiogenesis gene therapy in conjunction with coronary bypass surgery. *Circulation* 1998; **98:** I-321.

7. Gepstein L, Hayam G, Ben-Haim SA. A novel method for nonfluoroscopic catheter-based electroanatomical mapping of the heart. In vitro and in vivo accuracy results. *Circulation* 1997; **95:** 1611–22.

8. Kornowski R, Hong MK, Gepstein L et al. Preliminary animal and clinical experiences using an electro-mechanical endocardial mapping procedure to distinguish infarcted from healthy myocardium. *Circulation* 1998; **98:** 1116–24.

9. Kornowski R, Hong MK, Epstein SE, Leon MB. Electromagnetic-guided catheter-based intramyocardial LV injection: a platform for intramyocardial angiogenesis therapy. *Circulation* 1998; **98:** I-353.

10. Kornowski R, Fuchs S, Vodovotz Y et al. Successful gene transfer in a porcine ischemia model using the Biosense guided transendocardial injection catheter. *J Am Coll Cardiol* 1999; **33** (suppl A): 355A (abstr).

# Index